#8 IN THE SERIES OF
BOOKS YOU'LL
ACTUALLY READ

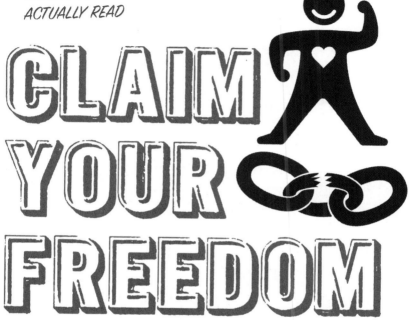

CLAIM YOUR FREEDOM

ANDREW EDWIN JENKINS

FORWARD & OILS INFO W/ DR. JIM BOB HAGGERTON

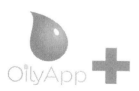 **+**

OilyApp

A BOOK YOU'LL
ACTUALLY READ ABOUT
THE FREEDOM SLEEP &
FREEDOM RELEASE KITS!

ISBN number = 9781077964501

#8 in the series of Books You'll Actually Read- go to www.OilyApp.com/books for more info about other titles.

Connect online!

Podcast-
OilyApp.com

Social-
www.Facebook.com/OilyApp
www.Instagram.com/OilyApp

Website-
OilyApp.com/Freedom for more info on this book

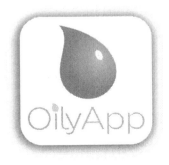

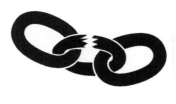

Contents

Part 2: The Oils

Part 3: Bonus Materials

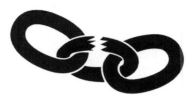

FOREWORD BY DR. JIM BOB HAGGERTON

Growing up I was always told I could be anything I wanted to be. That if I worked hard and did my best…I could accomplish anything. What my parents or my coaches or teachers never told me, or at least I didn't listen hard enough, was how much heartache and pain would be involved in that journey.

When my wife and I opened our first Chiropractic office in 2003 we struggled and worked our tails off to get it off the ground. But we loved it and never thought anything about it because it's what we had always dreamed we would do. The office exploded and we were busier that we could ever imagine and working from sun up to sun down…but still happy.

That all changed in 2011.

We had just had our second baby, Ellie, when all the wheels started to come off. The Lord saved our marriage from certain divorce that year, and we barely made it through that season. We thought for sure we had survived our roughest season, that we had "made it".

Then in 2014, after healing for those 3 years we were 33 weeks pregnant with Evans, our rainbow baby… and our journey got *even harder.*

Evans, unbeknownst to us, had Potter's Syndrome- a genetic mutation that affects kidney formation and lungs. He lived for 2 hours after delivery and we had to give him back.

We drove home that night with an empty carseat and no baby to hold and nurse.

That marked the beginning of serious hell for our family. The struggles we went through in our marriage were *nothing* compared to walking out losing a child.

Then there was more...

In 2017 while at a conference in Florida where I was scheduled to speak, I shattered my femur while doing a wave pool ride with my oldest son. Turns out, I had a benign tumor in my leg that had hollowed it out, making it so brittle that when I got in that ride and fell it just shattered.

I was in a wheelchair for over 10 months, and had to sell that practice we spend those long hours building when we first got married, because it took over a year to start walk ing again. I'm still rehabbing my knee over 2 years later.

Why does all of that matter?

Why bring it up?

What does that mean for you and why does this book matter?

It matters because all of us are going to go through hard things in life. The Bible actually promises us that we will. It says, "In this world you *will* have trouble" (John 16:33). It's a given.

The keys that got us through and keeps getting our family through so much hard are:

1. Not running from the pain and instead facing it head on

2. Drawing close to Jesus through it all (you can't do this alone)

3. Our warrior community of friends holding us up

4. Focus and vision and a purpose beyond just us

5. Essential Oils and their affects on our emotional centers

You're going to learn a lot about this process in this book. You're going to learn how to press into "the hard" and how to allow your body to work through the traumas you are either working through now or will face in the future. You'll learn things about your body that are key to be able to support yourself physically while you are going through hard things.

Above all you're going to learn what our family has learned through every hard thing we have walked through: *That there is HOPE even in your darkest day.*

Just don't give up friend. No matter how dark the night...the sun will rise.

Jim Bob

PS- A lot of people chase the sun, seeking daylight. In this book you're going to learn that one of the fastest ways to reach the light of day is turn and face the dark. Sure, that's counter-intuitive.

When you do it, though, you learn that the light actually begins coming towards you.

FOREWORD

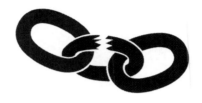

Intro: I Took a Psych Eval

Last Fall I did something I never imagined I would do: I took a psychological evaluation. A full one. The kind that has *hundreds* of questions followed by a sit-down interview with a licensed psychologist.

To say it another way, I *voluntarily* took one of those tests that cost several hundred dollars and can label you for the rest of your life.

Again, I *asked* to take it.

Here's why: smack-dab in my mid-40s I effectively averted the typical mid-life crisis by living a few tough years. Most people knew nothing of the trauma and trials I endured, but the pain was there. Every few months I spoke about pieces of my story from the stage at an event where I spoke, or I offered a glimpse inside my world via my podcast or some other venue where I taught. Looking back in the rearview mirror of my life, I realized I'd endured enough to knock someone off their feet and into the grave.

I mean it. The grave.

At one point several years ago. I actually contemplated suicide. Knowing life insurance policies like mine carry exclusion clauses which automatically negate the payout in cases of suicide, I *planned* the ordeal in my mind down to enough detail to make it emphatically *not* look like suicide at all.

Then I "got better."

And then- as often happens once you taste a bit of victory- the bottom of life fell out like the proverbial plank dangling over the edge of the pirate ship. Turns out, I'd learned to manage "fruits" without addressing the roots. (No worries if that sounds Chinese- I'll come back to the root-fruit issue in chapter 6).

I was regularly visiting a counselor when I took the eval. In fact, the eval was such a serious deal I needed a referral to get it. So, the PhD I was seeing did the honors.

That counselor happened to be the *second* professional I scheduled regular meetings with in the past 18 months. I abandoned the first after learning that although he presented himself as a licensed therapist he had no credentials at all. That's right, *zero*.

The first guy, though tender and kind, regularly over-stepped professional, ethical guidelines by providing legal advice and offering false wisdom which clearly landed far beyond his skill set. Ironically, I was referred to him by a friend of his who was- who is- a licensed counselor and, to my knowledge, also assumed he was credentialed. Kind-hearted and well-intentioned, he proved disastrous.

So, I found the second guy, Michael, someone whom I verified possessed the credentials and had enough history to help me move forward. After a few sessions, he assured me, "There's nothing wrong with you psychologically. You've just made a series of poor decisions. Some of those are understandable- not excusable, but understandable- in light of the circumstances you faced."

I mentally retraced the past few years, cataloguing each significant event in just a few micro-seconds.

"But I need to know if something is wrong with me," I told him. "I need to see for myself." Then- "If there isn't, OK. If there is, then I'm going to address it and get help. I'm not looking for a diagnosis, but I'm not trying to avoid one, either. I just want to intentionally walk in wholeness."

"OK. Let's do it."

With my insistence Michael referred me to Jeff, a licensed doc with a long list of professional credentials, numerous referrals, and his own history of helping people navigate the tough terrain of mental and emotional health.

I returned from speaking at Advance 10.0 in Minnesota on a Monday afternoon. I rushed my boys to Scouts to earn a Citizenship in the Community merit badge that evening, and then arrived at Jeff's clinic south of Birmingham the following morning at 7am for the eval.

Then I waited…

A few weeks later I received a phone call.

"Can you come in later this week?" It was Jeff. The doctor. I assumed he was calling to discuss the details of my evaluation with me, but he wasn't…

I contemplated not going for a moment. The first time I visited him for the eval, I went to the office where I was working with a nonprofit to create some tools on- get this- emotional and mental health. That morning, in the office, a runner served me with legal papers. I was being sued by someone who promised me just a few weeks earlier than they "weren't my enemy" and "could aways be trusted." What a whirlwind of a few days…

After a few moments, I came back to the present moment. I asked Jeff point-blank, "Do you have a diagnosis for me?"

"No, I don't," he said. "I don't have anything yet. I need more info from you. Your case is a bit complex, so I would like to interview you a second time."

A second time?

Most people simply took the test and then met with the PhD or PsyD afterwards. Not me. My story was so technical it necessitated a *second* discussion.

Was I that messed up?

I decided it didn't matter if I was or wasn't. **If the goal is to walk in total health, you turn and face whatever stands in your way and you move through it**.

NOT OUT OF RANGE

"Yes, sir. I'll be glad to come back," I replied. Then- "If something is wrong with me I want to know what it is so that I can address is and make it right. I'll meet with you as many times as you need."

In that moment I told myself, "Yes, great. I'm moving forward in the right direction. I'm going to get this figured out. *Finally*."

And, simultaneously, I thought, "Geez... I require more time and attention than most people. He's found *something*."

Turns out, he hadn't.

Well, that's technically not true. He didn't offer a formal diagnosis, but he did find *something*.

After another 90 minutes in his office, Jeff told me, "You're not out of range, so I'm not comfortable diagnosing you. That said, you do have some things that caught my attention..."

"What do you mean by *out of range*?" I asked.

"People assume that psychological disorders are either a *yes* or *no* proposition- that you're either a narcissist or you're not, that you're either a hypochondriac or you're not, that you're either an introvert or an extrovert, that you either have Post Traumatic Stress or you don't, that you either..."

"People see it all as black and white, as opposites? That's kinda how I do..."

"Yes, but it's not like that at all." He began drawing an imaginary scale- sideways- in the air with his hands. Then- "Think of it like this..."

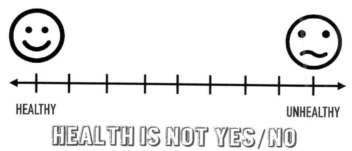

HEALTHY   UNHEALTHY

HEALTH IS NOT YES/NO

IT'S USUALLY A SLIDING SCALE... WE CAN MOVE IN EITHER DIRECTION

He explained that on one end of the line you have a totally healthy person and on the other end you have a completely unhealthy person- as far as that one issue goes. The MMPI, the standard test I took, measures for numerous psychological disorders, meaning you might be healthy in one area but unhealthy in another.[1] That is, the evaluation-instrument isolates different issues. And, the test is clever enough to tell whether or not you're lying or even "self-protecting" from the administrator of the test when you take it.

Brilliant, right?

Jeff continued, "Most people don't fall on either extreme. I mean, they don't fall off the one side where they're completely unaffected by something. In fact, that would be unhealthy. For instance, the extreme opposite of narcissism wouldn't be healthy, either- it would mean the person probably lacks self-worth and a healthy sense of their identity."

As I nodded in agreement, beginning to understand what he was saying, he continued, "But most people don't fall in the range where I- or any other professional- would diagnose them. There are a lot of people on social media using terms like *narcissism* and *gaslighting* and *abuse* who really have no idea what those words mean. In fact, many of the people who use those words the most are the biggest culprits..."

"I don't like it when people use those terms," I confessed. "They use them like grenades, and generally launch them at someone they had a disagreement with."

"That's only *part* of the problem," he said. "Another part of it is that most of the people who use those words completely misdefine them. They use them as 'hot

---

[1] https://en.wikipedia.org/wiki/Minnesota_Multiphasic_Personality_Inventory

words' without any true definition. Or, even worse, they supply their own definition. No one gets to re-write their own dictionary…"

He continued, "Another issue is that *because* they mis-define the words, and *because* they most often- you might even say *always*- use them in a negative sense- it keeps people who truly struggle with the issues from seeking help."

"That all makes sense," I told him. "People get understandably nervous when they think they might have a physical issue to deal with, but we don't attack them or assume inherent character flaws exist. With mental and emotional things, we automatically do."

"That's the other part of it. Mis-definition of it all makes people afraid of exploring an area in which most of us could benefit from a little help."

"How does this relate to me personally?" I asked.

"That's a good question. Your test came back and revealed a few things…"

"Like…"

"Well, first of all, you were a bit defensive."

"How so? I just answered a few questions with a pencil and paper before we had the interview."

"I know. The test showed that, though. There are questions built-in that screen that. You've been through a lot in the past few years, so this makes sense. It shows me that you're carrying some tension, some nervousness in general."

I thought for a moment, once again replaying various scenarios like the highlight reel of a horror flick for a few moments. I'd been a stress ball for quite some time, always bracing for when I was going to get emotionally punched again.

Then, I asked him, "What else…?"

"You're not diagnosable for *anything*, but I can tell you the things you probably struggle with…"

For the next 15-20 minutes I listened to Jeff graciously outline for me some of the deepest struggles I had- some of the same issues the people closest to me would understand once explained. Yet, I'd never heard someone detail them with such accuracy, with such honor, and with such tenderness.

"At some point, you had to crash," he said. There's no way you could keep carrying this weight. "Now that you're here, though, at the bottom, we can rebuild. And we can rebuild in the right way."

Jeff told me that **many people never seek help precisely because their cases aren't extreme enough to warrant a formal diagnosis. Yet, at the same time, they've been affected and wounded**.

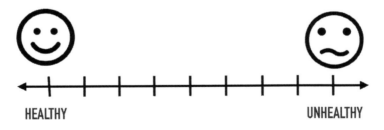

I thought about it. I'm not a psychologist, a counselor, or anything of the sort. In my mind, it all made sense, though. If you're looking at a scale of 1-10 and you need an 8 to receive a diagnosis, *what do you do if I you're just a 7?*

Or what if you're a 5- and are "only" halfway there?

A halfway broken bone is considered a fracture. A halfway "knocked out" boxer often has a concussion. A halfway working lung, kidney, or physical heart is… well… you might or might not even survive those halves…

So why don't we apply the same criteria to emotional or mental hurts as we do physical ones?

It means you go undiagnosed. And you, if you don't pay attention, you live with an undiagnosable struggle.

THE BACK-STORY

For years- probably a decade or more- my wife told me I needed to share my story with others.

"There's power in it. And healing," she encouraged. "Your words will set people free."

She felt certain that owning my story would set *me* free, too.

The problem was that my story was… well… *I didn't want to confront it.* I didn't want to admit what was there, buried somewhere between all the pages. **In order to share your story with others, you've got to admit that it is, in fact, *your* story.**

Parts of it were hurtful, painful, and self-incriminating. Parts of it were embarrassing. They were at the time, anyway.

I was afraid that in sharing it I would suddenly find myself *not* accepted but rejected. And, as you might imagine from a guy who reveals that he's "defensive" on a psych eval, relationships have been a fragile thing for me. I didn't want to deal with the "distance" with which people often inflict punishment when you disappoint them.[2] Rather than dealing with with truth- and moving into the light- I was content to live in the shadows.

As such, I got cozy there. I made my home in the dark for decades.

Trouble is, **there's no freedom in the places we hide-** *just a lot of fear.* Whereas we *think* that walking into the light causes fear and that living in the hidden places provides safety, the opposite proves true.

1 John 1:7-9 is a passage that's come to mean a great deal to me (NIV):

> *...if we walk in the Light as He Himself is in the Light, we have fellowship with one another, and the blood of Jesus His Son cleanses us from all sin. If we say that we have no sin, we are deceiving ourselves and the truth is not in us. If we confess our sins, He is faithful and righteous to forgive us our sins and to cleanse us from all unrighteousness.*

This promise in Scripture tells us that when we walk in the light (i.e., the "open"), two things happen: *cleansing and community*. Let me talk briefly about each, because this is profoundly true whether you ascribe to the teachings of the Bible or not. This simply works:

- **Cleansing**. Remarkably, 1 John is written to Christians- people who were *already* forgiven. That might cause us to think that cleansing is done- *because God sees us a clean*. Apparently, John's tribe needed an *ongoing* experience of the Lord's work in them.

---

[2] We'll discuss this in one of my favorite parts of the book, chapter 10.

The truth needed to move from information they held in their *head* to revelation they had experienced in their *heart*.

Something held them back from the freedom they were redeemed to experience. They needed an encounter which would allow them to *feel* in their heart the truth they knew in their head.

- **Community**. When we wear masks or live in those hidden places, we don't really know if people love us for who we are or if they love the false self we've projected. It's only when we walk into the open that we truly know each other. And it's only then that we experience the gift of true acceptance.

  John promised his friends that if they would walk into the light, the *right* people would fully embrace them.[3] They would no longer feel alone; they would experience the community we all so desperately crave.

For years I shared *only* the parts of my story I wanted others to see- the good parts, the places where I "had it all together." You may have seen those pieces of my story and applauded. Or "liked" it. Or "hearted" it. Or laughed. Or cheered.

The fact that I simultaneously struggled doesn't make those great parts less true for me any more than it makes the notion that your struggles make your highlights unreal, either. We're far more complex than we often realize.

In my life, those broken places occasionally surfaced. *After all, bad trees- or, at least, trees with chronic disease (or dis-ease)- bear bad fruits, right?*

---

[3] Note: some people *will* reject you when you walk in the light. It always happens. And it happens enough for us to question whether or not we should have really walked into the light. The right people, healthy people, will embrace you. Unhealthy people... *can't*. So they won't. That reveals more about them that it does about you, though.

The same symptoms continued resurrecting themselves in my life. Things like-

- Anger

- Lying

- Financial dishonesty

- A roller-coaster marriage marked by as many lows as highs

- Fractured friendships

- Trust issues (difficulty letting people close)

- Pride & posturing (spinning to make reality seem better than it is)

- Foreclosures (as in *three*)

- Bankruptcy

- Depression (it's hard to feel on top of the world when you live in the shadows and have so much clutter in there with you)

Whenever any of these things surfaced, I quickly "put out the fire," rationalized how the current circumstances created a *no-win* situation for me, and quickly hid the debris. Most people never knew *any* of this.

I always moved on with life, each time hitting a pause button on the chaos before watching an *even bigger* issue surface within the next few years. The more I prolonged dealing with the root issues and focused only on the fruits, the deeper those roots grew. They became stronger. They made their presence known.[4]

---

4 We'll talk more about this roots and fruit issue later in the book- in chapter 6.

Those issues always re-surfaced at the most inopportune times, too. Crisis is never convenient. In fact, trials often come during what seem to *already* be the most challenging times.

Over time I developed a fear that maybe one day I would have plenty of time to share my story, and that when I did I'd probably write it while in prison or share it with others at a rehab- from some place like the local mission two miles from my house, a place where guys learn about Jesus all day, spend their nights and Saturdays working at the nonprofit's thrift store, then get to visit their families for a few hours every other Sunday.

I know. Sounds weird. Looks weirder to actually type it.

NO SECRETS...

For years I was afraid of what might happen if I just shared my story. I was afraid others would shun me; I was afraid my wife would disown me. I was convinced that, in the end, it would just be me and my story, standing there all alone.

The truth is that the Accuser always accuses. Always has. Always will. *Long after the payment for sin has been made, he continues accusing.* Until his dying day, he'll continue escalating the chatter. Or, at least, *he'll try to.*[5]

Jesus knew this. As He approached Holy Week, He told His disciples, "Satan has *nothing* on me" (John 14:30).

---

[5] That's his name. See Revelation 12:10.

There was no secret thing the Accuser could pull from the closet of Christendom and toss into the middle of His story. There was no scandal, no hidden skeleton, no untold event.

Our lives aren't quite that pristine. Dig long enough, and you can find something on *anyone*, right? In my case, you wouldn't need to dig too deep or push too hard.

What's the path forward?

Ironically, freedom isn't found in burying the clutter deeper. That just takes the roots deeper and makes them stronger. No, freedom is found in bringing everything to the surface, right there where everyone can see it.

Sounds scary, doesn't it?

Again, **freedom isn't found in hoping that no one finds out. Freedom is found when there's nothing more to hide**, when the skeletons in the closet no longer have a stronghold on you (we'll discuss this more in chapter 9).

Of all things, the Holy Spirit showed me something about this while watching an "unholy" movie. And He highlighted the solution.

Here's what happened. One weekend I skimmed my Netflix "suggestions" and zoned-in on *8 Mile*, a film in which rapper Eminem plays Jimmy Smith, Jr., a young man who desperately wants to leave the boundaries of Detroit and move towards his dreams and destiny. Jimmy finds himself competing in a rap contest, the kind which pits two artists against each other.

The rules are somewhat strange: the rapper who insults the other the most wins. So, with the beat blaring behind them, artists accuse one another of their public flaws and hidden failures. It's basically *Devildom 101*.

During the final showdown, Jimmy flips the script, though.

Rather than insulting his opponent, *he focuses only on revealing all of his own faults*. He raps about his poverty, the fact that he's a different race, the truth that his girlfriend cheated on him, and that he got jumped and robbed a few days ago. In doing so, he effectively disarms the enemy, plundering him of his complete arsenal of ammunition. When Jimmy finishes, *there's nothing else that can be said*.

He concludes his routine, taunting his foe, "Now tell them something they *don't* know about me."

Eminem tosses him the mic. His only ammunition now stripped from him, the opponent grows more embarrassed by the moment. The opponent (Clarence) sheepishly hands the mic back over. There's nothing more to say. There's *nothing* left to accuse. Eminem plundered the enemy of his power by saying everything that could be said about him *on his own*.

To quote Jesus, "This accuser has nothing on me."

You can get to that place by living a perfect life that leaves nothing to accuse (like Jesus), or you can get there by unloading it all before the Accuser can. Most of have a trail of debris in our past, leaving us with option 2.

CLARIFYING WHAT IT MEANS

Jesus told Nicodemus, a Pharisee who searched Him out one night to speak to Him about "new life," that people who want freedom walk into the light, so that "their deeds might be exposed" (John 3:21). They don't hide.

And John told us- we just looked at it- that cleansing and community occur in that light (1 John 1:7-9).

Let's clarify what it means to "walk into the light." Most of us *don't* need to stand on a stage and "rap out" the highlight reel of our flaws, bearing (and baring) your soul for the masses. That's not the means I suggest you use to find wholeness.

I define walking in the light as this: *allowing the light to penetrate every dark corner and crevice of your soul, so that you might see what's there, deal with it, and find freedom.*

Walking in the light isn't so much a "public display" of your junk as it is a private penetration of the secret places. Oddly enough, our *hyper-sharing-place-it-all-on-social-media-for-everyone-to-se*e can actually mitigate against walking in the light. You can drop a note on social media and over-share parts of your life, effectively not sharing them at all.

How so?

Well, when you drop a post for a few thousand strangers to see, you off-load the info but you don't necessarily do anything with it. You just set it out there. You feel like you've done the tough work. The hearts and thumbs *seem* to confirm that you have. But you haven't. Most of the people who "like" and "heart" and even comment an "atta boy" know nothing of your story. They're just being… *kind.*

Transparency doesn't mean "disclose everything to everyone." It means you disclose everything to the people closest to you, that there are no secrets in *those* open spaces.

In his book *Culture of Honor,* Danny Silk communicates this truth with an incredibly easy-to-understand analogy. He writes something like, "If you're painting your house and you create a spill in the kitchen, you don't clean up the bedroom. You clean the kitchen."[6]

He adds, "You might alert people who walk into the kitchen that you've just mopped the floor, that they need to be careful they don't slip and fall." Then- "You wouldn't necessarily hang a *Slippery When Wet* sign in the garage or grab a megaphone and shout down the street about your accident to all your neighbors."

Makes a lot of sense, doesn't it?

The people who get to know are the people who *need* to know. And *maybe* a few others. But that's about it.

I outline it like this:

- **A few people get *everything*.** They get to know *every* secret hidden fault, flaw, and hurt. Nothing is withheld from them. This includes your spouse / significant others, your closest friends, and perhaps a few family members. This is an extremely small group of people.[7] They will graciously highlight your blindspots, encourage you, and empower you to live as the best version of yourself.[8]

- **Some people get *most things*.** That is, there are people who aren't in your inner circle who still receive access to significant parts of your story. For instance, I generally fill close business partners in on some of my recent clutter simply so they know where I've been.

---

[6] Danny Silk, *Culture of Honor*, https://amzn.to/2NchZ8c.

[7] For the men who attend the Advance, this is your "bus."

[8] I wrote about this in chapter 3, "Two Mirrors That Unmask Dysfunction," of *Emotional Wholeness Checklist*- the February 2019 release from OilyApp+. Go to page 40 in the book. More info at https://www.oilyapp.com/Feelings.

It gives them a grid whereby they can understand my current mindset and some of the decisions I make.

- **Many people get *some things*.** Over time, you might share parts of your life with others- with people in small groups, recovery centers, or even from a stage or social media.

- **Most people get *nothing*.** The reality is that although the situations you face are extremely important to you, they barely phase anyone else at all. They're busy clearing- or festering about- their own debris.

Lean hard on the first group, the small nucleus. And, when "their time" comes to deal with their own hard things (it will), hold them even harder and closer than they hold you.

The tendency in our culture is to hide- and then overshare. We tend to overshare with the masses, while hiding our hearts at a distance from those who remain closest to us. In a way, we confess- and get things off our chest but the relationships are never healed. We end up- get this- hiding behind a mask of *false* vulnerability. It's easy to do- especially when we get likes, shares, and comments from strangers about what we've walked through.

I know. There's some degree of irony in giving you that advice while I'm telling you parts of my story in a public venue. I mean, geez. I just put my stuff in print! It's different here, though, because I feel like part of my job- my calling- is to communicate and show others how to navigate their own terrain, so that they can do so on their own terms when they're ready. It's easier to do that if I can communicate something to the effect of, "Here, here's where I've been… and here's how I've handled it."

AND WHAT HAPPENS NEXT IS...

Somewhere I read, "You're in control of you." I've read that several times, in fact. Though it sounds true, it's a bit naive.

Here's reality: there are massive chunks of my story over which I have complete control. At the same time I, like you, live in real time and space where other people's decisions radically affect my future, the wellbeing of my family, and even my financial outlook.

Sounds scary, doesn't it?

I can choose to live as a victim of the circumstances I must endure, or I can choose to live above them- to live free- even as I walk *through* them.

Sometimes we're given a script we don't want to play. We find ourselves in a scene in which we adamantly don't want to be. We can still emerge stronger, though. And we will. We'll discuss the "how to" over the next few pages.

Now, the house-keeping details. This book consists of three parts:

- **Part 1 = Life is Good, and Life Is Hard.** We'll discuss the tough emotional territory of PTSD, emotional scars, and a concept known as Moral Injury.

  This part of the book, I feel, is strong enough to stand on its own.

- **Part 2 = The Oils.** We'll walk through the Freedom Sleep collection and Freedom Release kit from Young Living Essential Oils. Commit yourself to understanding and applying the concepts in Part 1 in order to get the maximum benefit from the oils.

In the same way that your essential oils are part of a healthy physical routine that includes nutrition, movement, and proper rest, emotional oils are only part of an "inner health" protocol.

In this book I advocate using Young Living's Freedom Sleep & Freedom Release kits. Since those two products are in such high demand, they regularly go out of stock. I'll provide you with some alternatives for times when that happens (see chapter 15).

- **Part 3 = Bonus Materials.** We'll discuss the financial cost of emotional health, I'll provide you with the chapter I think is the most important in the entire book, and we'll end with a self-check / assessment tool you can use to evaluate your own emotional fortitude.

That said, turn the page. Let's talk about perception and reality. We'll determine which one is more accurate. You'll discover that concept alone has a *ton* to do with mental and emotional health.

All the best,

Andy

June 1, 2019

PS- Although this is the 8th book in our series of "Books You'll Actually Read," this is the 3rd book we've released on emotional + mental (read: soul) health.

A few people have asked, "What's the difference between this book and the *Emotional Wholeness Checklist* (Feelings Kit) and *Healthy Hustle* (oils for work + life balance).

Here's my take-

- *Emotional Wholeness Checklist* talks about the importance of feelings- of embracing both the "good ones" and the "bad ones" and learning how to read what they say to us.[9] In doing so, we learn to let our feelings serve us rather than being hijacked by them.

- *Healthy Hustle* reminds us that many of the issues that wreck our souls have to do with our identity- of seeking to "fill" something in ourselves. When we get that right, we can live from a place of overflow rather than posture of constant striving.[10]

In this book we begin dealing with the grit left from the wounds of the past. We talk about the scars. We claim our freedom.

---

[9] https://www.oilyapp.com/Feelings

[10] https://www.oilyapp.com/HealthyHustle

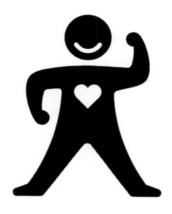

PART 1: LIFE IS GOOD, AND LIFE IS HARD

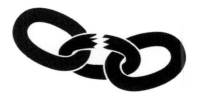

1. Live Inside-Out Not Outside-In

King Solomon said, "The righteous are as bold as a lion." The flip side, he wrote, is that "the wicked flee when no one pursues" (Proverbs 28:1).

When you get to the place Eminem found himself in that film I referenced in our intro, you can be *bold*. **When you realize your identity isn't found in the great stuff you've done *nor* is it defined by you at your worst, you can be *even bolder.*** You sense a humble, tender confidence swelling inside you- one not based on your perfection or lack of flaws but based on the notion that there's nothing else to hide. You've owned your story.

I remember the days of constantly looking over my shoulder, always wondering when life might come unzipped. Constant anxiety sucks.

When there are holes in your story, it's easy to hide. *You want to hide.* The problem, though, is that hiding makes things worse and more tense. Pressure builds beneath the surface. Sooner or later, whatever is inside surfaces.

King Solomon (a guy with a lot of clutter in the closet) also wrote, "One who covers his transgressions will not prosper, but whoever confesses them finds mercy" (Proverbs 28:13 TLV).

That's the magic thing we want: *mercy.*

Grace.

Freedom.

It's time to claim yours.

When we own our flaws, we allow grace to crash in and we simultaneously stop the enemy's accusations. The flip side is this: when we cover things, we push freedom to the side. It *always* remains available, but **it's impossible to grab hold of grace when you're clinging tightly to a mask of self-protection.** That gives the Accuser a field day.[11]

And it causes us to walk in more shame.

And timidity.

Take King David, for instance. He was Solomon's dad. 2 Samuel 11 records his affair with Bathsheba, the wife of one of his prized warriors.[12] David saw her bathing one day and summoned her to the castle.

He had his way, and she became pregnant. He tried *repeatedly* to cover the sin, culminating when he murdered her husband. If *he* was dead, everyone would just

---

[11] See also Proverbs 10:12, 17:9, 19:1. And, go to 1 Peter 4:8 and James 5:20.

[12] I'm not actually sure how accurate it would be to refer to this as an "affair." Those are generally two-way relationships. As king, he summoned her to come. Did she have a choice? We don't know.

assume the baby was his, right? After all, he wouldn't be around to tell them otherwise.

David (eventually) repented, but it seems he never fully dealt with the issue ("hiding" went deep in their family). *The episode marked him.*

Years later one of his sons raped one of his daughters (siblings by two different mothers, *but still…*). David refused to confront the sin (see 2 Samuel 13).

How could he? He'd *also* used his *own* position of power to sexually seduce a woman himself. He was seeing what he'd done play out right before his eyes. Even if he couldn't articulate why, he was hesitant. Timid. Un-lion-like. Un-bold.

Absalom, the full-brother of the harmed daughter, planned to kill David because he refused to address the sin. Absalom couldn't, though, because David wouldn't make time for him. He refused to go on the hunting expedition where Absalom planned to entrap him. So Absalom did the next best thing; he killed the perpetrator, the guilty half-brother (2 Samuel 13:23f.).

David wouldn't acknowledge *that* sin, either, though. He wouldn't extend his heart to Absalom even after that, resulting in a rebellion in the entire kingdom. David was forced to flee the palace.

You can't walk in your rightful role when there are parts of your story you're hiding. It's impossible to do so, because we're created to walk in the light. Because of that hidden sin, David refused to walk in his God-given authority.

Who was he to confront issues he saw in other people? He had the same ones which he refused to deal with!

LOOK INSIDE

Whereas we tend to look "outside" ourselves and focus on the externals, rationalizing that things will get better *for us* when things change *around us*, the opposite proves true. The *soul* is the internal thermometer that sets the temperature for the world around us.

John wrote, "Beloved, I pray you may prosper in all things and be in health, *just as your soul prospers*" (3 John 2, emphasis mine). Notice that he prays for prosperity in all things *and* in health. Yet, it seems that the soul is the measure of how much we can carry- in the prosperity of "all things" and in our total health & wellness.

We often "spiritualize" or "futurize" the blessings of God, believing they only matter in the after-life. When we do this, we reduce the stories of Scripture to allegory, effectively pushing the promises of God to a time and place where we don't experience the full benefits of them. John assumed we could experience these blessings *now*.

Notice, though, **your soul serves as the gauge for the experiencing the good things of life now.** Health. Abundance. (Yes, there are people who prosper in "all things" {financial provision} and health without getting the great work of the soul right. There are always exceptions to the rule. However, we shouldn't plan based on the exceptions.)

What's the soul?

Well, your soul is unique from your body and different than your spirit.[13] The soul includes your mind (your thoughts) and your emotions (your feelings).

---

[13] Notice Hebrews 4:12 says the Word of God helps distinguish the soul from the spirit.

Your soul is the thermostat for the world around you- and gets to set the temperature. It's not *just* a thermometer which simply reports what's happening. We often flip it the other way- and assume that we'll think and feel right when things outside become right. John pushes us in the opposite direction, though. He says that learning to think and feel right on the inside actually overflows to change the outside circumstances.

2016 was a difficult year- one of those years you definitely don't want to repeat. *Ever.*

2017 was OK. I thought I was in "recovery mode."

2018 proved to be the worst 365 day period I've experienced.

As I made my way through these strange seasons (in large part by the help of numerous "life rafts" people tossed to me along the way, often not even knowing they were doing it- just blessing us by being them, and gifting me in many ways with their presence at just the right moment), I decided it was time to go after the deeper issues and to seek healing from the things that had happened.

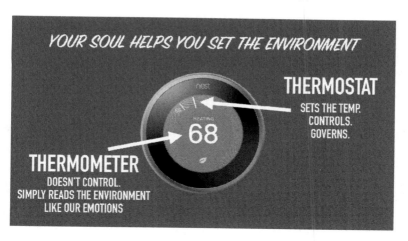

I studied several topics related to emotional, mental, and even spiritual healing. I studied in a different way than I had with most of my studying before. You see, as odd as it sounds, reading and writing can be somewhat of a "getaway" for me.

- I can *read* a book and actually "check out" of reality.

- I can actually *write* and do the same thing.

I know. Sounds surreal. You'd think mental work would be taxing, that it would drain me. I've found that my brain has greater stamina than my emotions, however. It's almost like when I do either (reading or writing) I can choose to step out of this world and into the world of whatever I'm reading or writing about. I can avoid and escape.

Over the past few months it finally dawned on me that this is exactly what I had done over the past few years. It's why, in the middle of stress and chaos, I can actually *choose* to work. And, I can do it well (i.e., some of the best material we have used at the men's Advance events was created during some of the most chaotic chapters of my life).

This season was different, though. Rather than studying and wrestling with *information*, I was actually digesting and wrestling with personal truths that I was hoping would bring about lasting *transformation*. This created a different sort of journey than I've taken with other concepts in the past.

- Information touches the head; *transformation adjusts your heart*

- You can remain emotionally neutral when you're studying information in the world of your mind (even if you are passionate about communicating it in a specific way); *your heart is never emotionally neutral*

- You can study information for a few minutes or few hours and then walk away; *your heart stays with you...*

My point is this: you've got to deal with the deeper issues on the inside in order to live well on the outside.

INSIDE-OUT NOT OUTSIDE-IN

At some point in my journey- a journey I'm still in, by the way- something clicked.

One day, while studying stress and trauma, I thought, "I'm going to list all of the things that have created high-level stress for me in the past few years."

I began listing them...

The list grew from the 2 or 3 I readily remembered to 5...

Then the list grew to 6...

And on to 8...

Then beyond 15...

Over *17* specific instances sat there, on that page, which could push anyone over the edge. I listed many of them in the intro. Yet, *here I am,* still standing.

The problem is that **even though *none* of those issues left scars on the outside, they all left internal marks.** Wounds. Hurts. Things which must heal.

If I broke my leg, I'd rush to the hospital and take care of it. It's an *obvious* wound. If emotional wounds actually left a mark outside of me- on my body, such that they were visible- I'd probably go to the doctor for that, too. The problem is that these wounds existed under the surface, though. Unseen, there was no urgency to deal with them. Yet, they inflicted the same damage a broken leg can- *and even more.*

Imagine me walking down the street. Your street, the one where you live. You look out your window and see me limp around with a dangling appendage, scars on my face, and jagged knife marks where I've been physically stabbed in the back.

You'd probably rush to my side and say, "Hey, wait! Let's get you some help!" You wouldn't even ask if I needed help. You'd know I do!

Those wounds are the emotional reality many of us carry. I've experienced it; you've probably experienced it, too. (While we're at it, let's just confess that we've probably dealt some of those emotional blows to others, right?)

Yes, we've got to do the tough work of the soul. We've got to deal with the unseen scars, the hidden wounds. **If you *don't* do the tough work of the soul, you'll continue interpreting the future in light of the past- in light of the things you've done wrong and the things done wrong to you.**

This means that I'll continue walking in hurt *and* I'll continue hurting others rather than being an oasis of radical grace. So, the healing must happen.

Apart from inner healing, you'll never set the thermostat from inside your soul. You'll continue looking outside yourself and just assume the temperature is correct. Remember, thermostat- *not thermometer.* That is, even though you're affected by the climate around you it doesn't get to control you- even when it presents the circumstances in which you find yourself.

That said, turn the page. In order to live this "inside-out" thing, there's a is simple truth we've got to get right, something about how we perceive reality.

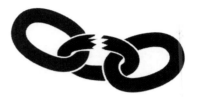

2. Spoiler Alert: Perception ≠ Reality

You've probably heard the phrase "Perception is reality" a few times.

As correct as that statement sounds, it's just not accurate. Perception *might* be reality, but it might not be. Perception *might just be the way you view things.* Again, perception *might* be reality, but it *might not* be reality at all.

Let me show you…

Let's say I write a big number 6 on the ground. I write it in large 6' tall letters, using it to denote the number of biological kids I have who have a birthday *before* Salter, my youngest kid, who just celebrated his *sixth* birthday, has another- his seventh. In other words, my *6* is laced with numerous objective facts.

For the sake of illustration purposes, you see me from afar and walk my way.

"Why did you draw a *9* on the ground?" you ask.

"I didn't. I painted a large *6*." Then, I explain everything I just wrote.

You don't understand. Looking at the number from your unique vantage point, you actually have the audacity to correct me (I know, it's just a humorous analogy, OK?). "If Salter is *6* then why did you write... a *9*!"

I tell you that *you* have it wrong. "I didn't. I made a *6*." I step over and trace it with my steps. "See, it's clearly a *6*!"

"Umm, no. You just walked out a *9*," you reply.

We go back and forth, back and forth, round and round, over and over...

Question: *Who's right?*

From one person's perspective the number on the ground is clearly a *6*. From the other's... it's a *9*.

Obviously.

A politically correct cartoon from which I ripped this example actually said something like, "See, what you see depends on where you stand?"

The cartoon inferred that both people saw reality accurately. But, both people *can't*. While there are a lot of things in life in which shades of grey are the norm (i.e., think back to my psych eval and who gets diagnosed as opposed to who doesn't), most things are actually *concrete*.

I drew a *6*. Salter *is 6*. It doesn't matter where you "stand" on that issue, those facts don't change.

Your interpretation of the facts might change, but the facts don't. In other words, your perspective- your perception- might *not* be reality.

THAT WAS THEN, THIS IS NOW

For the past 18 months I've worked with veterans- particularly in the arena of mental, emotional, and spiritual health (all three areas are unique yet simultaneously connected in ways I'll outline in this book). These valiant men and women regularly communicate how things they experience *now* are often colored by things they experienced *then,* back when they served.

"I don't like the 4th of July," one man confessed. "At night when everyone begins shooting fireworks, it seems excessive. One or two might be OK, but the ongoing barrage sounds *exactly* like the mortar fire that came at us in Afghanistan. I'm obviously proud of our nation and the 4th, but I can't do those sounds. I go inside, close the doors and curtains… I usually turn on some music or watch a loud movie."

Another vet offered, "I still lurch when I hear a car backfire or hear any other abrupt sound. My body automatically jolts, and I look to take cover."

A third warrior told me it wasn't just sounds that affected him. One day, as we sat at my kitchen table looking at some essential oils, I handed him a bottle of Frankincense. He immediately scooted his chair back, his face froze, and he gently cried…

"You alright?" I asked.

"I just need a moment," he said.

I nodded, remaining quiet.

A few minutes long later he "came back" to the moment. "I'm fine," he whispered. "That smell was *everywhere* in the Middle East when I was deployed. I saw a lot of hard things there, and smelling this transported me back to where I was when all of that was happening."

Here's my point: in each of these instances the mind and the emotions- that is, the soul- pulled someone out of this moment and thrusted them into another one. **They began interpreting- or, perceiving- the present in light of the past**.

Fireworks aren't mortar fire.

Cars with troubled engines aren't guns.

My kitchen table isn't a camel driver's tent in the middle of war-torn Iraq.

In the same way your perception assured you I sketched a *9* on the ground instead of a *6*, their perceptions *assured* them of something that wasn't true. In other words, perception wasn't reality.

I learned from the veterans that PTSD (Post Traumatic Stress Disorder) is a lenses that causes people to see the world in certain ways- often misperceiving the way things really are. **When the mind and emotions create false impressions that jerk us into an alternate reality- one we *perceive* to be true rather than one that *actually is* true- it might be an indication that we're still dealing with past trauma**.

Turns out, this is true for many of us. A lot of the things we see *might* be related to past hurts, past internal wounds that we carry around. Left unchecked, those wounds can become the filter where by we view the entire world.

POST TRAUMATIC STRESS IS...

Now, my goal isn't to diagnose you- anymore than it was to receive a diagnosis for myself. In fact, I'm not a licensed therapist or clinician or counselor or any other thing. Ethically, then, I *can't* diagnose you.

But I *can* throw some concepts out there, highlight a few things, and then encourage you to do some self-exploration. That's what this section of the book is about.

That said, notice the American Psychiatric Association's definition of *Post Traumatic Stress Disorder*. (And, remember, like the licensed professional told me, you don't have to be diagnosed in order to be affected by something.) PTSD is-

A psychiatric disorder that can occur in people who have experienced or witnessed a traumatic event such as a natural disaster, a serious accident, a terrorist act, war / combat, rape or other violent personal assault.

Here's a graphic to help you remember it-

POST TRAUMATIC STRESS

"A psychiatric disorder that can occur in people who have experienced or witnessed a traumatic event such as a natural disaster, a serious accident, a terrorist act, war/combat, rape or other violent personal assault."

SOURCE = AMERICAN PSYCHIATRIC ASSOCIATION

I want to highlight two things from the definition above-

First, you may or may not have experienced the situation firsthand in order to affected. That is, something might have happened to you or it could have been something you saw.

For instance-

- Getting shot *might* cause Post Traumatic Stress.

- Watching someone else get shot *might* have the same effect.

Or-

- Being physically or verbally abused *might* cause PTSD.

- Living in a house where someone else was abused *might* have the same effect.

I highlighted the word *might* in my examples above, because- as you'll see- we all respond to the same potential stressors in different ways.

Second, there are a variety of scenarios that can cause the stress.
Emotional trauma can come, according to the APA's definition, from a storm, a car (or other kind of) accident, war, or any kind of physical abuse. Furthermore, their definition includes that open-ended phrase "such as," showing that those are only *examples* of things that, again, *might* cause PTSD. Any stressor has potential.

Again, remember (I know, I keep repeating this) you don't have to have a diagnosable disorder in order to be affected. Even though you might not have a formal diagnosis, you could still experience- or see- any of these events (or others "such as" them) and have your own form of invisible scars.

THAT WAS THEN AND THIS IS NOW

The first night I taught this concept to a group of veterans something dawned on me.

"You're not abnormal," I said. "You're normal." Then- "You're responding to events completely in line with your training. You've been trained that when a loud sound occurs that it's either mortar fire or machine guns. The present action of wincing when you hear fireworks and the pop of an engine is consistent with your past experience."

One gentlemen shook his head in affirmation. He saw it.

Then another.

And yet another.

Then the entire group.

It's not crazy to take cover when mortar rockets start flying. Or when bullets whiz by. Or when someone has flipped their lid and is about move into full blown rage, coming against you physically. Or when _____.

Fill in the blank. You get the idea. **Those are normal responses to events that- by their very nature- create traumatic wounds and demand a defensive posture.**

I knew I was connecting with the group, so I continued, "The problem is that you're responding to a different normal than the current normal. You're perceiving something, based on your experience, that's no longer true. In other words, your perception is no longer reality."

Then one of the attenders made the connection for us all. "That's exactly what it means to be triggered, isn't it?"

> # We might mentally or emotionally react to a *different* event than the one we are experiencing.
> ### *(PERCEPTION CAN BE REALITY)*

I thought about "getting triggered" and what that means. That guy suddenly made a concept that's well-worn and tossed around so often that it's virtually lost any semblance of meaning radically understandable. He helped us comprehend what it means to find yourself *triggered*.

"Yes. That's a great point. **To get *triggered* means you suddenly find yourself firing off in a certain direction based on some perceived threat from which you need to protect yourself.**"

"Yeah," one of the women added, "and we don't even think of it as being triggered unless it's a false alarm. If it's a real threat, it's a threat that you responded to in a healthy way."

"I think you all are onto something." Then, after a few moments of processing what they were saying- "You're really helping me understand some things I've experienced but haven't had language for before. Thank you."

Think about it. Then look back at the quote box on the previous page:

> We might mentally or emotionally react to a different event than the one we are experiencing.

That's what it means to be *triggered*. **The emotional- or mental- unhealth comes in the fact that we're responding in the wrong time, in the wrong place, making it the wrong thing for the moment.** In other words, we're "triggered" by something in the present that powerfully connects us to the past- not to the present.

Or, to say it another way, we're responding to something besides the now.

Or, there's a disconnect between our perception and our current reality.

> # Your response would be completely appropriate in a different time + location.

One of the warriors concluded, "So in the same way we trained our brains before, coaching ourselves to look for mortars and bullets, and to actually face them while others take cover, we've got to train them again to actually hear fireworks and engines."

"I think so," I told him. "And I think you can."

How does it relate to me and you?

Turn the page and we'll talk more.

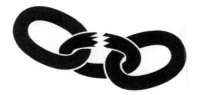

3. The Goal = Health

Emotional health (in fact, health in general) isn't so much about what's wrong with us as it is about what's right- and walking into what's *even better*. In our medically-driven, diagnosis-prone Western world we've been conditioned to look at problems rather than seek solutions. And, we've been trained to "fix issues" rather than walk in wholeness.

This applies to emotional health, too.

Whenever I speak to a group about emotional wholeness, many people assume that my goal is to convince people they have emotional scars which need healing. That's simply not true.

Therefore, my goal is *never* for people to "get a diagnosis." Or even to take a psych eval. I'm simply honest about my story because, well, that's my story.

My goal is to help people walk in freedom. *Period*.

If a diagnosis or even just an evaluation is the path to freedom, so be it. Many times, it's not, though. In fact, *most* of the time simply having the information is enough.

That said, let me show you something about Post Traumatic Stress.

BEEN AROUND AS LONG AS PEOPLE

Many people think PTSD is new. Turns out, it's not. In fact, it's been around for an incredibly long time. In fact, it's probably been around as long as people have been.

For sure, the actual term *Post Traumatic Stress Disorder* didn't come into popular usage until after Vietnam.[14] However, historical evidence indicates even warriors in ancient times suffered its effects.[15] In fact, though it may have been identified by different terminology, we see examples throughout history.

- During the Civil War it was called "soldier's heart"

- During WWI & WWII, it was called "shell shock"

- During the Korean and Vietnam wars, it was known as "combat" or "battle" fatigue

You've probably heard these terms before. Each one references the same internal struggle.

As it pertains to military service, it is important to note that its effects are not unique to American soldiers. PTSD is experienced among those on *both* sides of a conflict.

---

[14] See *Warrior Hope*, Bob Waldrep & Andrew Edwin Jenkins, pp31f.

[15] It is clearly evident warriors experienced it in Biblical times, for instance.

POST TRAUMATIC STRESS *IS NOT NEW!*

* **Biblical times**
* **Civil War = "soldier's heart"**
* **WWI, WWII= "shell shock"**
* **Korea & Vietnam = "combat" or "battle" fatigue**
* **Today = Post Traumatic Stress Disorder**

Again, "soldier's heart" and "shell shock" are concepts which have been around for decades.[16] I remember hearing each of these terms when I was a kid, generally in reference to an older veteran in our church. The terms were most often used anecdotally, pointing to someone who had trouble adjusting to social norms.

Thankfully, our perspective on PTSD has changed. Shannon Polson, a Clinical Social Worker featured in the documentary *Honoring the Code*, notes that its formal recognition as *Post Traumatic Stress Disorder* did not occur until 1980 when it's entry into the DSM-3 put PTSD and the field of traumatology on the map.[17] According to Polson, this was the first time it was ever formally acknowledged, lending credibility to the field.[18]

Some people disagree as to whether or not we should use the word *disorder* when referring to PTSD / Post Traumatic Stress Disorder:

---

[16] See *Warrior Hope*, Bob Waldrep and Andrew Edwin Jenkins, pp53f.

[17] DSM = *Diagnostic and Statistical Manual of Mental Disorders*. This provides the criteria, the standard, professionals use to diagnose, treat, and prescribe.

[18] To stream this documentary free go to www.WarriorHope.com/HTC.

- Some people feel the word *disorder* carries a stigma that may hinder people from seeking treatment.

- Others point to the fact that psychological diagnoses fall on a spectrum (like we discussed earlier in the book) and that you can be greatly affected by something and not "qualify" for a diagnosis.

- Still others remind us we don't label other common human health concerns- broken bones, the common cold, or even cancer- as disorders. We simply diagnosis them and then move forward with treatment protocols.

Generally, people opposing the use of *disorder* prefer substituting the word "injury" or the word "symptom" or they omit a fourth word completely.

I recently watched an interview with a Democrat Presidential candidate who is a veteran. When asked about trauma he experienced in war, he referred to "PTS."

When you hear the terms Post Traumatic Stress Symptom or Post Traumatic Stress Injury, the same soul wounds are being addressed. This is certainly an important discussion, but as PTSD remains the term used for diagnostic purposes in the current DSM, it's the identification I'll use in this book.

WHAT PTSD LOOKS LIKE

Experts generally agree there are four broad categories of symptoms that help them to recognize and diagnose PTSD properly. Note: you can experience multiple symptoms concurrently.

1. **Hyper-vigilance**– can't relax and has difficulty concentrating and sleeping. Everyday sounds, such as a backfiring car or fireworks may cause anxiousness or even elicit a trained response, such as duck and roll. They may tend to sit with their back to the wall in public places in order to be aware of the environment before them.

2. **Re-experiencing symptoms**– nightmares or flash backs where they feel like they are back in that traumatic situation. Certain sights or sounds may trigger these memories of that danger or stress.

3. **Avoidance symptoms**– does whatever they can to avoid anything that reminds them of that trauma. They may want to avoid riding in a car, watching certain movies, or being around certain people– and avoid talking and even thinking about the hurtful memories.

4. **Negative feelings**– may be extremely depressed, have angry outbursts, or just can't control their emotions. They may be fearful of others or are not able to trust other people.

You might read those four points and think, "Those responses seem fairly common."

Turns out, they are. Depending on this situation, you may have experienced each of these symptoms before. I have.

This is one of the reasons I advocate walking in health far more than I encourage seeking a diagnosis. Besides, a diagnosis means nothing if you don't follow through with the intention to live healthy and whole.

That said, the result of feeling these symptoms generally takes two opposite approaches, depending on the makeup of the person:

Some people fight. Some people choose to turn and face a direct threat. They may become aggressive and launch a retaliatory assault- even against perceived (yet unreal) threats.

You may have done this yourself or you might have experienced this being done to you before when someone "pops off" verbally in a way that's disproportional to the actual threat they're experiencing. "The best defense is a great offense" is the mantra of survivors who choose to fight.

Others take flight. That is, they avoid the conflict altogether, protecting themselves by removing themselves from the situation.

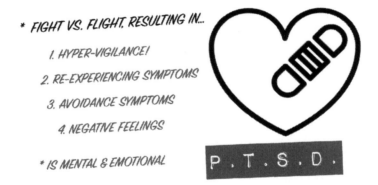

* FIGHT VS. FLIGHT, RESULTING IN...

1. HYPER-VIGILANCE!

2. RE-EXPERIENCING SYMPTOMS

3. AVOIDANCE SYMPTOMS

4. NEGATIVE FEELINGS

* IS MENTAL & EMOTIONAL

P.T.S.D.

Some people might choose to fight in some situations while electing to take flight in others. Often, it depends on the type of perceived threat, as well as whether or not they feel responsible for others who are present (example: I might respond to a true threat of a car-jacker differently if I was alone as opposed to if I had my daughters in the car with me).

IT'S COMMON

A lot of people think PTSD is rare. That's another misperception. Turns out, it's actually quite common.

What's *uncommon* is the formal diagnosis. In order to be diagnosed, people must meet specific criteria.

In the back of this book you'll find a self-evaluation / Post Traumatic Stress test (chapter 17). When I was writing the book *Warrior Hope* (for veterans), my coauthor and I located the test on a VA website.

The version of the test in this book lists 8 criteria related to PTSD. At the time I began researching it, *veterans were required to meet all 8* in order to receive a formal diagnosis. In addition, three more factors came into play-

1. The trauma had to be linked to a specific event which they could recall to a licensed professional, *and*

2. At least one of two additional "specifications" had to be met. That is, the person had to either *de-personalize* the issue (i.e., "this didn't happen to me," as if they're living in a dream world) or they had to *de-realize* it (i.e.,, "none of this is real"). *Furthermore,*

3. At least six months had to pass between the onset of the issue and the date of the diagnosis. Even if symptoms occurred immediately, time needed to lapse to prove that the issue was now an ongoing soul wound.

In my mind, there are a couple of red flags with these additional qualifiers:

First, many times it's difficult to hitch soul wounds to a specific event.
That is, traumatic feelings are often the result of *a series* of events. For instance,

- If a soldier survives multiple deployments and takes gunfire numerous times but only feels the emotional pain *after* she slows down enough to catch her breath and assess what happened, *how can she necessarily pinpoint which precise moment birthed the trauma?*[19]

- If a spouse is verbally berated by his wife such that gaslighting and name calling and psychotic control occur on a monthly (if not weekly) basis for decades, *is it any "less real" because he can't determine the exact moment it began to feel less like a regular marital spat and more like one-sided, heavy-handed abuse?*

Because of the nature of life and the changing dynamics of human relationships, in most situations it's mind bending– if not impossible– to determine which precise instance of trauma is the straw that broke the camel's back.

Second, humans have an uncanny way of white-washing the past, of looking through the rear-view mirror with rose-colored classes. We tend to minimize the emotional hurts we feel, because of two facts:

1. Time *does* heal a lot of wounds (or, at least, it heals them to *some* degree), *as well as*

2. Someone always has it "worse" than us, thereby causing us to minimize our pain (we'll circle back to this notion in chapter 7).

---

[19] This exact scenario occurs in the final episodes of season 2 in the television series Seal Team. A former Navy Seal cannot pinpoint the precise moment his trauma occurred, even though all of the symptoms are present and verifiable. As such, he is ineligible for treatment.

As a result, depersonalization and de-realization are real issues that occur even when people are healthy.

Third, finally, waiting 6 months from the onset of traumatic injury until a diagnosis is received is, on one hand, a positive step, but it's short-sighted. It's rarely a good idea for someone to receive a diagnosis after just a few days. The wounds are too raw to completely assess.

At the same time, we clearly *don't* wait for 6 months to label physical wounds. When something is amiss, we address it. In large part this is because, particularly when it comes to physical hurts, the goal is often to "get well" rather than living in the diagnosis.

A REALLY HIGH BAR

That said, those are lofty criteria to meet in order to receive the formal label of Post Traumatic Stress. Since there are only 8 criteria, you must score "perfect" on the test in order to receive the diagnosis.

And maybe they should be case. After all, we're looking at a label someone will carry with them for quite some time- a moniker that often lands on job applications, school forms, and every health questionnaire you'll ever complete in the future.

Let's say you *don't* score perfect, though. And, for the sake of argument, let's say you *don't* want the diagnosis. You *don't* want the label. That's probably most of us...

But let's say you emphatically *do* want to walk in health + wholeness. That's probably most of us, too…

Are you less affected because you score a 7? Does that mean you shouldn't address the emotional hurts that caused you that much (but just short of diagnosable) internal pain?

I've read and re-read that test dozens of times. I've looked at it as I've listed to veterans and business partners and friends share their stories. I believe that most of the people who read this book probably score 5-6 on the test. They're not diagnosable for PTSD any more than the average person on the street is diagnosable with cancer.

But not having cancer doesn't mean we don't walk in perfect physical health any more than not receiving a PTSD diagnosis assures we're emotionally whole. **There's always room for greater levels of health- especially when we're not afraid of labels and we've embraced the notion of total wholeness as the goal.**

Again, the goal isn't to receive a diagnosis (nor is it to necessarily avoid one). The goal is complete wholeness. And the reality is that, in some sense, precisely because life is both good and simultaneously hard, most of us have soul wounds.

Where do they come from? And how do we identify them?

We'll discuss it that issue more in the next chapter.

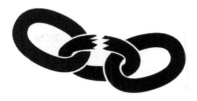

4. Self-Protective Self

In January 2019 I wrote *Emotional Wholeness Checklist*, a book about feelings and the importance of recognizing them in ourselves.[20] The premise is this: ***all* of our feelings- both the ones we typically consider to be "good" and those we often consider to be "bad"- are important. Emotions are to our souls the same thing physical sensations are to our bodies.**

Think about it…

- When we feel physical *pain*, we understand that something is wrong. We could be sick, we might be tired, or we might be in danger. The "bad" sensation highlights that something is "off."

- When we feel physical *pleasure*, we know that things are (most often) right. The euphoric feelings of post-exercise or post-sex bliss communicate to our bodies that we are satisfied and safe.

Turns out, our emotions *can* work the same way. We just have to learn to read them before we react and then manage them before we make a mess of things. Joy and

---

[20] https://www.oilyapp.com/Feelings for more info.

happiness and other positive feelings tell us that we're in a good place. Emotional hurt tells us we're not.

As I was sorting through all of this, trying to locate language whereby I could understand and express my ideas in that book, I knew I wanted to speak with Dr. Benjamin Perkus. Dr. Perkus (DP) has 20 years of clinical psychological experience. That's his professional training. To be clear, whereas I can't diagnose people, that means he actually can. He has the training, the earned credentials, and the wisdom only time (a lot of it) can bring.

PROFESSIONAL + PRACTICAL + PERSONABLE

One day DP told me, "I loved my craft, I never envisioned myself leaving it, and always thought I'd write a book about my practice some day. I just wasn't sure when and how."

Turns out, he worked extremely close to home. On his front porch, in fact. A few years into practicing psychology, he and his wife "closed-in" the porch, creating an office near the front door of his house where he saw clients.

An innovator, DP ventured into ground-breaking techniques when he began practicing two decades ago (i.e., EMDR, tapping, etc.). So, when he was first introduced to essential oils in 2001, he was open to the possibilities.

He and his wife became distributors with Young Living Essential Oils. Over time, as they had success using the products as part of their overall health and wellness routine (and invited others to do the same) their essential oil biz grew.[21]

DP says, "I was was living a dual life in the good way, doing *two things* I equally loved."

From his office on the front porch he was a practicing psychologist, a good one. From his kitchen table, he was an oiler. People visited his home for one or the other constantly. Sometimes, many times, for both.

Fast forward to 2015. Young Living held their annual International Grand Convention at the Gaylord in Dallas (I remember it well, as I spoke twice at this event!).

DP says he spoke with his upline one day and confessed he was "torn" between his two professions. He didn't want to give up either. He saw the power and efficacy of each- and the need for both of them. In effect, each one actually enhanced the other, making him more effective on both platforms. As a Platinum distributor in Young Living with a growing biz, how could he and his wife choose?[22]

His upline leader, Connie McDanel (a Royal Crown Diamond, the highest rank in Young Living) encouraged DP to "create a tool."

He decided the tool would be a book. Again, he always thought he would write one. He'd just assumed it would be related to psychology- not essential oils.

---

[21] Listen to his story on episode 43 of The OilyApp+ Podcast at https://www.OilyApp.com/blog/43.

[22] Go to www.YoungLiving.com/IDS for more about the income potential.

By his own admission, "I had no idea it would involve *both*- and that it would be in everyday language that *anyone* could understand- even if they didn't know know psychology and even if they didn't know much about the oils."

At that point in his story, DP had been traveling (at Young Living's invitation) to teach about memories and trauma and other things he taught via psychology. And, he'd begun using essential oils to empower people towards healing. It was *all* part of his presentation.

In April 2016, almost 9 months after that enlightening convo with Connie, he decided he to jot a few notes for his eventual book while on a flight to Singapore. He returned and decided to churn out the book in time for the AromaSharing event (read: vendor hall) at next convention, slated for mid-June! He had 60 days to go from *potential* to *print* to *press*. The book was completed, people wanted training to help others with his technique, and the entire movement known as AFT (shorthand for "Aroma Freedom Technique") was launched.[23] Quickly.

"I hadn't even *thought* about certifying people to use my methods at that point," DP told me. "After that, I knew I needed to figure it out. So we did, and the story continues unfolding."

As we do with each monthly class for OilyApp+, I wrote the *Emotional Wholeness Checklist* book, taught the class, and then created graphics and other content relevant to the overall theme of soul health and wholeness. Since emotional health was a significant part of my personal focus during that season, I landed there for my content creation for about two months.[24]

---

[23] https://aromafreedom.com for more info.

[24] Like a mentioned in the intro, this is when I cranked out *Emotional Wholeness Checklist* and *Healthy Hustle* in back-to-back months.

I wanted to dive deeper, though, as this was a topic that and continued resonating with me for the past 3 years or so, since that difficult 2016. Having been dealt traumatic blow after blow (many of them the results of my own actions; others the results of others' actions), I decided to pause and explore this area more. Turns out, I have a "job" that offers me that freedom and flexibility. So...

- I hosted two podcast conversations with Dr. Perkus.[25]

- I contemplated AFT certification- something I decided I'll do in the near future when the right time presents itself.

- I scheduled a Zoom call and put our OilyApp audience in front of Dr. Perkus, where they could hear how his technique works, ask him specific questions about his AFT, and then actually experience his technique firsthand.[26]

After telling me the story about how AFT was born, DP explained how it works.

Now, this book isn't about the AFT (you'll need to buy his book to learn that). But, there are three powerful truths DP told me on those podcast interviews and during the Zoom call that have everything to do with claiming your freedom. And that is why I include this part of his story here.

DP told me, "There are three facts about human nature."

Then he outlined the three...

---

[25] Go to episodes 43 and 44 of the OilyApp+ podcast. Search with your favorite podcast provider, or go to https://www.OilyApp.com/blog/43 and https://www.OilyApp.com/blog/44 . Perkus leads a "reset" during the second talk.

[26] https://www.oilyapp.com/AFTZoomReplay to watch the video replay of this talk- given by Dr. Perkus.

DESIGNED TO EXPLORE + MORE

"**First, we're designed to explore and grow**," he said. "This happens from the day we're born. Infants begin crawling- and even poking into areas they shouldn't."

"Yeah," replied. "It seems like little tots are always trying to poke forks into electrical sockets, jump into cabinets, and push the bounds of what's permissible. It's almost like you tell them not to do something…"

"… and then that's what they do," Perkus concluded. Then- "It's because we're created to explore."

"What's the catch?" I asked.

"That leads us to the second point. **We're designed to explore, but we're also created to learn from our experiences and then- now, get this- to avoid pain in the future by creating inner rules**."

"What do you mean?"

"Well, the inner rules our are ways of coping with the fact that some of our experiments hurt us. Some exploration is good, some exploration is bad. You lose some of your innocence as you venture into new territory, causing you to start playing it safe."

"When my kids were little," I told him, "they all used to *love it* when I tossed them in the air. They would- every single one of them- run up to me, stretch out their arms, and ask me to *chunk* them up and catch them. So I did…"

He laughed. "Ever drop one of them?"

"*Never*. But they all started getting nervous about being thrown 'high in the sky,' as some of them called it, about the age of 3 or 4. They used to *beg* me to do it, then they- almost overnight- all grew *terrified* of it. I never understood why, because no one ever even came close to getting dropped."

DP had some insight: "By then they had all learned to walk, though. And they had fallen. They had begun to ride bikes and probably taken a few spills."

"So they knew they *should* be afraid of heights," I concluded. Then- "That makes sense. I was tossing them 8 or 9 feet in the air. So that helps me understand it, now."

"OK," Dr. Perkus said. "Now that you understand *that*, apply it to other areas of life. You learn not to cry, because you do it one day and someone belittles your feelings. Or you get stage fright because someone makes fun of your singing voice. You learn not to trust people because a friend shuns you at the playground…"

"Oh, my," I replied. "I've already got a list that's a mile long of things I continue learning *not to do* even today…"

"Well, most people do. The problem, though, is that we don't even think about these rules we create. They're often kept hidden from our conscious minds. They just become our default mode of operating, almost like we're on auto-pilot."

I thought back to my discussions with veterans- about cars backfiring and fireworks. And to convos I had with friends who had "yellers" and "screamers" in the house when they were growing up. Or people who got "frozen out" when they revealed something about which they had a disagreement with someone… how they all created these "rules" in order to avoid future pain, because they'd all done a bit of exploration and found out that life, though it's good, is hard. The world isn't always safe. Getting *triggered* is the logical outflow of these protective rules.

"I've got a confession," I said. Then I hit him with it, half-joking. "I'm not an 'animal person.' Used to be. Back when I was little. But I just figured out why I stopped being one…"

"You created a rule about animals, it seems."

"Yeah. I loved dogs. Always had one. Then one day I went to my friend Daniel's house and had a run in with one. His dog, Snoopy, was sleeping in the cockpit of an old fighter jet they had in their backyard. It was just the windshield. That was Snoopy's house."

"Was Snoopy a dog that looked like the actual Snoopy?"

"No. He was a bigger dog. A big greyhound. A grey-blue color. He was normally pretty chill, but when I walked over to him- I was only 7 or 8 years old- I woke him up and startled him. He lunged at me. And snapped. It legit scared me. I started crying, even though he never bit me."

"And you still don't like dogs today?"

"It's not that I *dislike* them. It's just that, well, I've kept my distance from them since that run-in with Snoopy. Yeah. I guess have a hidden rule."

"Most people do the same thing in their own unique ways. **We learn most of what we know by experience.** We do this with hot stoves. And heights. We make rules that say don't touch hot things and don't go too far away from the ground. Like your kids did."

I thought for a moment and then continued, "I imagine **we also learn to avoid certain things in relationships- we dump others before we get dumped. We hide our true selves. We guard our hearts. We stop being vulnerable. We withhold affection when we're afraid it won't be reciprocated. We stop trusting.**"

As we talked, I sketched the "three facts" into my black Moleskine journal.

THREE FACTS ABOUT HUMAN NATURE

 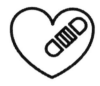

1. EXPLORE + **2. PAIN** + **3.RULES**

WE'RE DESIGNED TO DEVELOP & GROW AS WE EXPLORE THE WORLD AROUND US

SOME EXPLORATION CAUSES PAIN- WHICH WE WANT TO AVOID IN THE FUTURE

WE CREATE RULES- OFTEN SUBCONSCIOUSLY- TO HELP US AVOID FUTURE HURT

"We do *all* of that," Dr. Perkus said. "Here's what you need to see, though. The rules fall into two categories. They can be functional rules or they can be dysfunctional rules…"

He described them as you might imagine:

Functional rules actually help us. They keep us from pain in *healthy* ways.

- Rules that keep us from touching hot stoves are helpful.

- Rules that keep us from walking down dark alleys at night, swimming in the ocean alone, or walking into oncoming traffic are healthy.

- Rules that caution us to take an Uber if we're going to drink at dinner serve us.

You get the idea. Rules- even the ones we don't think about- can serve us.

Dysfunctional rules hinder us. They keep us from progress in *harmful* ways.

They're based on perceptions of reality and are often consistent with our past experience. Think back to the mortar fire and bullets.

(By the way, sometimes these rules have a basis in past reality, sometimes tghey don't. Sometimes, they're consistent with our past perceptions only.)

INTERNAL RULES- FRIEND OR FOE?

TYPE OF RULE	IS A...	RESULT
Functional	Friend- helps us	They keep us from pain in healthy ways
Dysfunctional	Foe- hinders us	They keep us from progress in harmful ways

"The problem with these rules," Perkus clarified, "is that **our brains don't distinguish between which rules are functional and which ones are dysfunctional. Our brains simply create rules and follow them indiscriminately.**"

"Alright," I said, "you mentioned there were three facts about human nature..."

YOUR HIDDEN AGENDA

"Yes. The first is that we're designed to explore and grow. The second is that we experience pain when we do. Third, our brains create rules to help us avoid pain…"

"And," I interrupted, "some of those rules make sense, some of them don't."

"Right. **That leads us right into the bigger issue as it relates to trauma and healing. Here it is: *we hide those rules from our conscious mind*.**"

"What do you mean we *hide* them?"

"I mean you might not even know that the rules is there. Or, to say it another way, you might have a mental block to something and not even know the block exists."

"So I may have an agenda and not even know what it is?"

"Kinda. You might have an agenda that's hidden even to you."

As I pondered mindsets and thinking patterns and the *perception-isn't-always-reality* tension, Perkus offered me an example: "You've probably seen a dog with an invisible fence…"

"Yeah, there's one down the street from my house. Whenever I run, he darts from the porch and makes a mad, rabid dash right at me. Used to freak me out because of my past experience with Snoopy. Until I figured out that dog would get shocked if he touched the sidewalk. He simply barks loud and toes the line all the way across his yard. I kinda taunt him now, to be honest…"

"You might need an AFT session for dogs only," he said. We laughed, then he continued, "When that dog was young, he was trained *not* to cross that barrier- or he would be shocked. Today, the dog *could* actually get to you and bite."

"Oh, my!"

"I don't mean to burst your bubble, but he *could*. In time, the trainer removed that barrier that *would have and certainly did* jolt him, yet even now dog remains in his yard." Then, after a short pause, he asked, "Why does he do it?"

"Because one day he went exploring- *Fact 1*. But, he experienced a bit of pain- *Fact 2*. So he created a rule- *Fact 3*- don't step off that grass, lest he get electrocuted."

"Right. No more exploration and growth for the dog. He's not even aware the shocker is gone. He just obeys the rule without thinking about it as his default mode of living. **We often obey our own hidden rules as our default- regardless of whether they're functional or not.**"

"Like the elephant being held by a rope?"

"Yes. Or like the person being held back from their dream, the person afraid of success, the person stuck in a negative pattern. Somewhere, if they think back through it, they have some hurt… so there was a basis for the creation of the rule."

"But now there's not?"

"Maybe. Maybe not. But if something is holding anyone back from their destiny, it's certainly worth exploring."

SOUL MEMORY / MUSCLE MEMORY

Last week I made a quick day-trip to the Nashville area for an online project I've been working on for a few months. On the way back to Birmingham I stopped in

Huntsville to eat dinner with my parents. While splurging on Red Robin's bottomless fries (me) and the never-ending salad (my dad), some of these concepts started crystallizing in my mind. *There's nothing like a few hours of windshield time alone to mentally process some things.*

Dad offered me the regular (and always sincere), "What are you writing right now?"

I was midstream into writing this book, so I explained the previous few chapters.

"Did you see the NBA finals?" Dad asked.

"No. I watched *zero* minutes of NBA basketball all season..."

"Oh, well, Steph Curry is an example of what you're writing about. Except it's muscle memory, not emotional or mental or soul memory. He practices his three-pointers over and over until they're almost automatic. When he releases the ball, it's almost a *given* that it's going to go in the hoop. It doesn't matter how many defenders jump on him, how much they get in his face, how bad his balance is at the moment, or even if he gets bumped..."

"...At some point his muscle memory just kicks in. That's why he gets paid big."

"Yes. Golfers, too. A lot of the guys on the PGA circuit hit the same drives over and over. They repeat them. *Ad nauseum.* More than I've ever seen. But, when the crowd is there and the stakes are high, they put the golf ball exactly where they want it to go. Muscle memory. It's a real thing."

"And so is emotional, mental, soul memory. **We live forward based on what's happened in the past-** *even if the present is nothing like the past.*"

I wondered what would happen if a basketball player practiced his shot wrong for, let's say, *a few thousand* reps. Practice *doesn't* make perfect. Practice makes, well, *more of whatever you practiced*.

- Practicing the wrong thing creates the wrong muscle memory.

- Believing (and even feeling) the wrong thing creates the wrong *soul-memory*.

In other words, **if you follow those hidden rules too often for too long a duration, you may need to release and then intentionally rewrite them. But that requires identifying the rules that are even there.**

Shooting a game-winning three-pointer is actually quite a feat when you face a handful of almost-seven-feet-tall-Herculean-athletes charging you. The situation creates a heap of tension.

But the championship game doesn't have to be on the line to experience such drama. Just about anything in life can do the job.

For instance, many of us actually know what we want to do, what we desire in life:

- We crave a thriving marriage- but need to face some tough convos in order to get there

- We desires to grow a large, prosperous business- but need to "put ourselves out there" and lead others in order to do so

- We imagine ourselves going back to school- but need to make some scheduling things happen before such is a possibility

You get the idea. There are probably a lot of important things you want, things just on the other side of an invisible fence that you're afraid might shock you.

But, and this is the kicker, **many of those hopes and dreams stand in contrast to what's safe.** Those things are our version of the game-winning three-point shot, made while falling backwards and jumping amidst galloping foot traffic while hearing people in the stands cheering for us and against us at the same time. **While all this occurs, our rules continue informing us- even if we're unaware of them, even if the boundaries are no longer in place.**

It may be that we have the wrong soul-memory, right?

In fact, as you began envisioning what any of those "victories" or "dreams" might be for you, your mind might have begun flooding with negative thoughts almost immediately.

Sometimes, we "go to war" with our thoughts. Doing so often creates an internal tug of war, a true struggle. So, we push our way through until we, inevitably, hit a wall and stop. The "stop" often reinforces a rule- an invisible one- we hold in place. And, a bunch of rules strung together often create a script, a story line we begin living, all as a means to manage our environment and protect our self from pain.

In the next chapter we'll talk more about this script, as well as what we can do if we don't like the string of scenes in which we find ourselves.

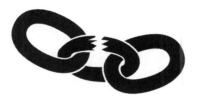

5. The Story We Tell Ourselves is the Reality We Sell Ourselves

In chapter 2 we talked about perception- and how that perception often becomes our reality if we're not careful to separate what we think we see from what we actually see. Then we discussed internal rules- mental agreements we make with ourselves (often subconsciously) which help us sort and maintain some degree of personal safety as we navigate life. **In the same way elite athletes thrive from muscle memory, we often navigate life in both good ways and bad ways from *soul-memory*.**

In this chapter, I want to push that idea a bit further, because **soul-memory is built in small everyday encounters. But, the overall impact of these encounters, over time, becomes exponential.**

TOLD WHAT TO SEE

In the book *Sway: The Irresistible Pull of Irrational Behavior* (now, think about that title!), Ori & Rom Brafman write about the effects of pre-existing beliefs and how they effect our ongoing belief patterns- even when confronted with new information to the contrary.[27] (Remember, Dr. Perkus told me some of our self-created internal rules are functional and some are completely dysfunctional.) The Brafmans write about a visiting lecturer, a guest teacher at MIT. As an experiment, the teacher lectured 70 economics students at the prestigious university.

Now, you've gotta think- if anyone is not going to be irrationally swayed by something, it's going to be this bunch of smarties, right?

Well, *wrong.*

All 70 students were given a bio on the visiting professor. The bio was a page long and detailed the prof's accomplishments. The students were instructed to review it *before* listening to the lecture.

Here's the set-up:

- Half of the students received a bio that said the guest teacher was "a very warm person."

- The other half received a bio that said the prof was "rather cold."

That's it. *No differences otherwise.* The students all listened to the same lecture at the same time, and were then asked to grade the professor.

The results were, well… revelatory.

---

[27] Find the book on Amazon at https://amzn.to/2Yeo9pE.

- The half who read the "warm person" bio wrote how great the teacher was. He was funny. He made them laugh. He told great stories and made things applicable. He actually made economics exciting!

- The half who read the "rather cold" bio said the teacher was aloof. He was self-centered. He was rigid, inflexible, and boring. Oh, and he was formal. Stiff. Lifeless.

Did they not sit through the same lecture at the exact same time?

Of course they did.

What happened?

Quite simply this: the students saw what they already believed to be true.

How so?

Their perceptions were all front-loaded. They were told what they were going to see.

As a result, reality or not, that's exactly what they saw.

WE SEE WHAT WE'RE LOOKING FOR

Many times we see what we've already decided we'll see. In other words, seeing is believing, yes. But, often, believing is seeing.

See how that works?

- If you're looking for reasons why you'll get a bad outcome, you'll likely read everything through that lenses.

- If you believe you're going to succeed, that you're going to have a great outcome, you'll (likewise) look at everything through that lenses.

This is especially true when past trauma is involved. If you're looking for mortar fire or bullets or people to shun / hurt / abuse / take advantage of you, etc... well, you'll likely see what you've already decided to see.

Internally, **your mind will subconsciously kick into over-drive, scanning the universe for hints and clues to back up what you've already determined to be true. Then, *that* will become the grid whereby you view reality**.

(And every now and then reality will actually match your perception completely, thereby giving your false impression enough credibility to continue.)

I decided to try this theory out one summer while at the pool on vacation. I often give my kids a "challenge" when we're swimming. Something like "do 10 flips under water." Or "catch a pass behind your back while jumping into the pool." It's become an expected game we play every time we're at the pool.

"What's the challenge for the dollar?" they ask.

(I often reward all the winners with a dollar they can blow on video games when we go eat pizza, use to load up on candy from the grocery store, or do something else whimsical.)

On this trip, I had already asked them to swim sideways across the pool- *there and back*- underwater, holding their breath. No one had even *tried* it yet. They had all *assumed* it was impossible. They stood there in the pool fretting about how it couldn't be done.

Their mom leaned to me and said, "This is a great time to give them a pep talk..."

So, I ran an experiment about beliefs and perceptions and how they alter reality. Particularly those big subconscious ones- the ones that tell you that you might die.

"Kids," I said, "turn around and look around the pool. I want you to take 5 seconds, while I count out loud. Count how many *blue* things you can find."

I began counting backwards down from 5...

Quickly, they began counting up from 1, each of them rushing to find *blue*.

- Some noticed the *blue* sky

- Others noticed a *blue* tool shed

- Someone insisted the water should count, since it was a light *shade of blue*

- Another spotted a toy that had *some blue* in it

After 5 seconds I stopped them. Then I asked, "How many *green* items did you see?"

"We were counting *blue*," they told me.

Each of them.

They posted their numbers to prove it. Some had 6. Most had 3 or 4.

"It doesn't matter," I reminded them. Then, "I want to know how many *green* items you found."

"None," one of them finally told me.

"*None?*" I asked. "You have the grass all around this pool and at least a few hundred trees."

"We didn't see *green*," they said. "We were looking for *blue* things."

I explained the gig to them. I showed them how I had set them up.

"You found blue," I said, "*because that's what you were looking for.* Even if there is infinitely more green here to be found. In the same way, you assumed you couldn't make it across the pool, so you looked for reasons to prove you couldn't do it."

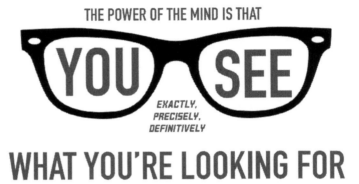

THE POWER OF THE MIND IS THAT

YOU SEE

EXACTLY, PRECISELY, DEFINITIVELY

WHAT YOU'RE LOOKING FOR

I reminded them of what they told me about the swim-

- It's too far

- We're not strong enough

- We're too tired because we stayed up late last night and have been playing all day

- We're too little and the pool is too big

Sometimes we believe something because we see it. Most of the time, though, we see *because we already believe what we're looking for.* And those are two different things.

Notice what Proverbs 23:7 says about this: "As a man thinks, so is he..."

Turns out, they *all* made it across the pool after our short coaching session.

Why is a picture worth 1,000 words?

Because if you see it, even in your mind, with your thoughts, you can tap into it... and then do it!

What have you seen before that you need to "see again"?

TIME FOR A REWRITE

We actually have the ability to stand "outside ourselves," observe, and edit the narrative. That means this: *your mind can observe what your brain is doing, what it's thinking, how it's responding* (sounds odd, but if you've ever thought through a few "if-then" scenarios then you know *exactly* how this works).

Dr. Caroline Leaf calls this **Multiple Perceptive Advantage, a way of viewing our lives that allows us to stand "outside" of ourselves and view reality**

from multiple angles. MPA makes mind renewal possible. Every human has it- you just need to develop the skill set to leverage it.

That means this: **since you can see how you're responding and reacting in the moment, you can actually change that response… in the moment.**[28]

And that means this, too: **if you can string together a whole bunch of these moments, intentionally, you can change the entire story arc of your life.**

That is, we can change the script we read to ourselves.

You can change the narrative.

Don't like the way things are going?

Rewrite your story.

Don't like playing the tragic hero?

Do a recast.

Rather give your "hero" certain gifts, talents, relationships, places to go and things to see…?

Time to rebrand.

Once you understand the power of the mind… and how it literally creates destiny, some of the most popular Bible verses make even more sense. Things like…

- "Take your thoughts captive" (2 Corinthians 10:5)

- "Be transformed… by renewing your mind" (Romans 12:1-2)

---

28 This concept is the crux of my *Emotional Wholeness Checklist* book.

- "Be anxious for nothing…" (Philippians 4:6)

- "Think on things that are pure, lovely, good…" (Philippians 4:8)

When we really believe that we can do these things- that we *can* take thoughts captive, that we *can* transform ourselves by proactively recreating what's in our minds, that we *can* choose peace over anxiety and stress, that we *can* select the object our our thoughts- we begin to see just how powerful we are.

BACK TO THE PERCEPTION ISN'T REALITY TANGO

It's easy to look at where we find ourselves in life and grow disheartened. We look at our progress- or lack of it- and feel we might be further along towards our dreams and goals if we were in a better place.

A few weeks ago I was pulling a few clips from a documentary produced by a nonprofit where I do some writing and teaching. I came across a segment I clipped from the documentary *Honoring the Code* to post on social media.[29] I'll tell you about the film later, in the chapter about Moral Injury (Chapter 9, "More Powerful Than PTSD").

Mary Neal Vieten, a Navy Corps Commander and PhD / Clinical Psychologist who served numerous soldiers returning from Iraq and Afghanistan reminds them that, "You didn't leave trained for combat as an elite soldier at the top of your game and

---

[29] Stream the film at WarriorHope.com/HTC.

then come back certifiably insane or crazy. **The things you endured are hard. They mark you. It's normal to be affected by them.**"

Or, to say it another way, "**You're not foolish because you have these internal rules that have created this story that you've lived.**"

Many of those internal rules are natural responses to real issues you've faced. And, in many senses, they're the things that got you through. They helped you survive. **But now you're in a different place. As a result, it's time to scrub the rules that no longer serve you, so that you might live a better version of your story.**

A few pages ago I referenced Dr. Caroline Leaf's book *Switch On Your Brain*. In that book she reminds us that some of the clutter we've got to clean up isn't the result of random things we experienced; a lot of it is the result of choices we made. Even then, though, we can step "outside of ourselves," use the MPA to look around, and make course corrections. In her words,

> It's important to make a distinction between who you truly are- the real, multifaceted, unique you- and the person you have become through toxic choices. [30]

So let's own that, too. You see, the reality is that-

- Sometimes we suffer because of what others have done to us (we're the victim)

- Sometimes others suffer because of what we've done to them (we're the perpetrator, which leaves wounds on them and an entirely different set of wounds on us- equally calling for a rewrite)

---

[30] See *Switch On Your Brain*, p45

- Sometimes we suffer because of what we've done

We can courageously own all of this, because we're not defined by the past and we're not stuck in the beginning (or even middle) of our story, regardless of how we got there. **There are still pages to (re)write, still a script to be lived.**

And the story we tell ourselves is… and will be… the reality we sell ourselves.

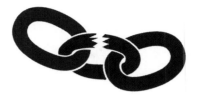

6. Roots & Fruits /
Causes & Symptoms

You might have read the previous chapter and thought, "Oh. He just inferred we can *easily* rewrite the script- that if we don't like the story we're living, we can just sprinkle in some new characters, change the scenery, add a few *power-ups*, and then move forward."

No so fast. You can't create a script overnight. Not a good one, anyway.

Here's what I mean...

Every few months someone asks me, "How long does it take to write a book?"

"What do you mean?" I ask.

"How many hours? Or days? Or what do you do? Do you just sit down and start until it's done, or..."

When I studied writing as an English Major at Samford University, I learned Jack Kerouac famously hammered out *On the Road*, a novel which defined a generation, in three weeks on a continuous reel of paper.[31] That approach generally doesn't leave space for reflection, for editing, and for course corrections- three things life requires that hacked-out novels might not.

I usually tell people, "It takes what it takes."

Then, "I work best when I can jump into the project and stay in it, kinda getting lost inside the words and pages…"

Re-scripting your story, your life, is much the same. **Unwriting old rules and thinking patterns, determining what responses are needed as opposed to those which are no longer needed… adjusting your soul-memory… none of those are instant "fixes."**

Let me pull back the curtain, share with you a piece of my story, and highlight what I mean. This is about to get *raw*.

OWN THE HARSH REALITY

"What are you seeing about yourself? Let's label it. Not to limit you and box you in but to get a starting point. **Truth is freedom. If we can define where we've been we can always navigate from there to where you're designed to be**."

Sitting in my attic office I was speaking with a life coach via Zoom. For the previous few weeks we had walked through the hurtful parts of my story. Like you and I discussed in the previous chapter, some of those parts were the results of things

---

31 https://en.wikipedia.org/wiki/On_the_Road

that had been done to me; many of those parts were the results of my own actions. Either way, though, I was responsible to take stock of where I was, own my story, and step forward responsibly. We were beginning to look at what moving forward looked like.

I answered him quickly. I began pushing through the list of things I was seeing about myself immediately. Words that usually scared me rolled *readily* from my tongue.

After a few moments, I concluded, "I don't know of anything else. I've laid it all out there. I can't think of anything I've omitted."

"Addiction," he offered. "You haven't mentioned the word *addiction*. I would like you to explore that. Maybe- *just maybe*- you need to look at yourself in the mirror and add this one, too: *I am an addict.*"

When he mentioned *addiction*, I began to see everything about my story through a new lenses. You see, I understand what addiction looks like. No, I hadn't see it in myself. I'd seen this one *clearly* in others.

For almost a decade I worked with addicts- the kind you conjure in your head when you hear the word *addiction*. The people hooked on heroine, LSD, marijuana, and other drugs. Alcoholics. Chain smokers.

It's easy to look at *them* as say, "Oh, yeah. *That* is an addict."

I watched person after person- or, let's just label it like it is, *addict after addict*- walk through the door of various transitional housing facilities and shelters where I worked for almost a decade. Residents generally moved through the first 30-day phase of the programs without any incidents. They found gainful employment. They reconnected with families who became confident enough in their progress to begin visiting them the 1st and 3rd Sundays of the month. They began laughing and smiling and speaking about the future in hope-filled ways.

Then- many times on the very night they received their first paycheck- they threw it all away for a night of some combo of sex, drugs, and alcohol. It's almost as if they became a *completely different person*- a person seeking to sabotage their hopes and dreams rather than fulfill them. **It was as if they had their own unwritten rules that subconsciously tossed them into that bad-outcome script, no matter how hard they fought for the good-outcome version**.

I worked in the field long enough to watch the same people recycle themselves through different programs. Like a revolving door or a merry-go-round, it was a predictable loop we could chart:

- Check-in to one ministry center or rehab for help

- Make meaningful progress

- Crash out

- Come to the senses and decide to go to another facility

- Make more significant, visible progress

- In short order, crash yet again

- Rinse, dry out, repeat entire cycle

It was surreal. I listened many of their stories firsthand, the very hour they wandered through our front doors.

"What brings you here?" I often asked.

"Wow! Things have got to change. And this time they will. I must jump off this roller coaster." Many then told me about the seemingly endless rinse-and-repeat spin cycle they were on...

For sure, many of them *did* change. Their lives were *transformed*.

But many of them didn't. Their lives weren't altered in the least. Eventually, four or five years down the road, some of that second group came back to our program- many times forgetting they had ever been there before.

That cycle *could* continue almost indefinitely- especially with so many residential recovery centers in our city. When it did, it always baffled me.

Why would the couple living on the family wing of that rehab program I ran for 7 years, choose to get high again? They knew a failed drug test would most likely mean they would lose custody of their kids for good and that at least one of them might very well go to jail.

Why would this man who finally held a steady job, guaranteed on-time transportation to and from work each day, and a forced savings plan which insured he would graduate our program with $5,000- $7,000 in the bank for future expenses to begin his life anew just toss it away to live on someone's couch- just so he could "drink one or two beers" every night after work?

I watched the cycle of devastation claim person after person. For years, I tried to figure out why they acted like they did, why some internal switch flipped and they suddenly began acting... *dangerously*.

I decided the issues weren't practical at all (i.e., "If I could just explain to them on paper or rationalize with them, illuminating the path forward.").

I decided the some of the issues probably centered around internal rules people created (i.e., "I'm not worthy of success or meaningful progress").

I decided some the issues were cover-ups for hidden pain, that they were coping mechanisms to block out the sound of "fireworks" or "backfiring engines" or some sort of other present thing being misperceived in light of the past.

In other words, the issues were deep.

DEEP LIKE ROOTS, NOT SURFACE LIKE FRUITS

I used to think addiction was a "fruit," that it was simply bad choice people made. Turns out, it's not.

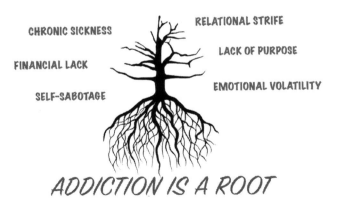

We could teach people about relationships, purpose, emotional health, or any other thing we saw manifest in life. We could instruct them on the healthy version of those things, but those are all fruits. That is, they're all symptoms (read: results) of our hearts being attached to the right place.

When our hearts are whole, relationships work. And we find purpose. And we're emotionally stable. And we don't self-sabotage. And we have enough. (Think back to the thermostat-thermometer analogy in chapter 1.)

I assumed addiction was simply one of those bad fruits people needed to be taught about. If they only knew better, they could do better. Or so it seemed.

Addiction is a root issue, though. Not a *fruit* issue. To kill it, you've got to destroy the roots, not just keep plucking off bad fruit. Unless the stuff inside changes, the fruit always returns.

It might take a few weeks (read: first paycheck) or it might take a few years (example: recycle yourself back to the same rehab you've already been doing, not even remembering you've already been there), but the fruit always returns. To change the fruit, you've got to deal with the root.

Now, I also assumed addiction centers mainly around substance abuse. Or porn.

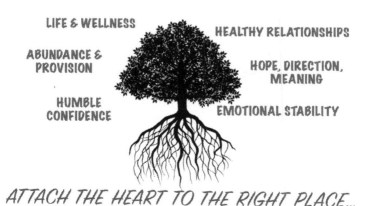

LIFE & WELLNESS　　**HEALTHY RELATIONSHIPS**

ABUNDANCE & PROVISION　　**HOPE, DIRECTION, MEANING**

HUMBLE CONFIDENCE　　**EMOTIONAL STABILITY**

ATTACH THE HEART TO THE RIGHT PLACE...

But addiction, a root, connects to other soil as well. **Addiction happens when we attach our hearts- for whatever reason- to the wrong place. And when we do that, bad fruit always emerges.** In order to see meaningful fruit grow in a consistent way, we've got to attach the heart to the right place.

All that said, I'd seen addiction firsthand. I watched amazing stories of redemption and recovery unfold right before my eyes, and I watched people choose lives of sheer hell. I even wrote the 12-step curriculum we used at The Village. I shot an entire video series for it.[32]

SOMETHING IN COMMON

Though I never made the connection between what I taught and what I lived before hearing the label *addict* during the Zoom counseling session, I suddenly saw something new. I could see the *same patterns* in my own life. My heart had been attached to the wrong things.

When I look back at my life through the lenses of *addiction*, things complete sense:

- In the same way *those addicts* would go to extreme measures to find their "high," so also would I. (At that point I still had to determine precisely what my drug was. I knew life had been spinning out of control. I was held things together on the surface, but I was sinking.)

---

32 You can watch it free at www.TheNextBestStep.info.

- In the same way *those addicts* spurned family and friends, sacrificing them on the altar of their addiction, so also had I.[33]

- In the same way *those addicts* sacrificed their health and sleep and rest, abusing their physical bodies to chase their addiction, so also had I.

- In the same way *those addicts* covered-up their actions and stole in order to fuel the addiction, so also had I.

- In the same way every addict I ever met who was stuck in their addiction denied having a problem, so also had I...

I've mentioned it before... for years I wondered if I might end up somewhere like *those addicts*, walking those halls, attending those classes, getting shuttled to and from work every day, having a chance to see my kids every 14 days in 2-4 hour time blocks or while on a weekend pass as I spent the rest of my time working on the deeper issues- issues at the time I couldn't even fathom were there.

"Go to some meetings *for addicts*," my coach told me. "Get online and see what's out there in your area for things like you've struggled with."

It's amazing what you can do with a label when you're not afraid to confront the hard truth. In looking at my story, I consistently chased two things:

1. Drive ministry forward (whether it was the church where I was on staff, the nonprofits where I worked, or some other project to which I was committed)

---

33 Think: workaholic.

2.   Please my wife- or keep her appeased. That is, don't rock the boat.
Save the peace.

On the first count, it was the ministry and the perceived success of it that fueled my ego, providing me so much of the personal validation I craved. And, It was "acceptable" to work long hours- because it was "the Lord's work." I could always rationalize that life and death issues- eternity and souls- were at stake.

One of my friends, as he resigned from our ministry years ago, told me, "I can't work here anymore." He added, without being asked, "You do the right things, but you often do them in the wrong way. It's not *what* you do, it's *how* you do it."

Short-cuts. Long hours. Insane schedules. Control. Bull-dozing people so I could finish my latest project.

That summarized the first point above perfectly. I was doing great work, but I managed it *like an addict*.

On the second count, I had to come to terms with the fact that I desperately wanted my wife to respect me, to think I was valuable, to believe there was greatness inside of me. I lied and covered up to avoid arguments with her I knew we'd have if I owned my un-success, my failures, or my inability to provide something she wanted. I continued my charades, in large part, to create a sense of security and even abundance for her. I wrongly looked to her for the years of validation which (in my mind) I never received. As a result, when she was pleased with me, I was ecstatic- on Cloud 9. When she was displeased, I was depressed.

As a result, I did everything I could to keep her pleased with me- even if it was a fake "pleased," measured against an impossible standard.

In some sense, all men want to please their wives. I'm convinced that women have no idea how much shame they inflict on their men with eye rolls, bickering, and verbal reminders that he doesn't measure up. Though I felt the tension that's common to most men, I went too far in trying to impress my woman.

Those were my "highs," they brought me a sense of value and purpose and meaning. They were a means of escape.[34] They covered the hurts of the past and filled my emotional tank.

NOT AFRAID OF LABELS

All that said, I attended a Celebrate Recovery meeting.

As I left that first evening, one of the leaders handed me a small book to take home and read. I flipped through it while grilling burgers one evening, then finished reading it as a sat post-dinner on our front porch.

I learned that 2/3 of the participants in CR actually don't have a substance or chemical addiction. Most of them are just seeking total wholeness, to see radical grace infuse their life in a way that nothing else in the world can. Notably, most of the issues are related to emotional wholeness- that one area I was beginning to learn is a significant one we often overlook.

Although that's not the impression we have of addiction, that's the reality. **Many of us attach our hearts to the wrong things (in large part, because of past hurts and pains we're seeking to soothe). We live from undisclosed hidden rules- in an effort to avoid pain. We cover that pain with**

---

[34] See Craig Groeschel's book *Hope in the Dark*, p83, for more about this.

addictions, false-fillers which can never eliminate the void. The result is bad fruit, bad fruit which returns perennially.[35]

I can't begin to tell you how many times I "killed" bad fruit in my life. "This is it," I repeatedly told myself. Then, to use the language from the title of this short book, "I'm finally free."

But I wasn't. Not for long.

Often, seemingly out of nowhere, bad fruit returned. When it did, it often grew back stronger and bigger, making it even more difficult to pluck off the next time.

Maybe you've been there, too, experiencing the same thing.

At some point, it made me think, "Dang. Maybe I'm just a bad tree. Because good trees bear good fruit and bad trees bear bad fruit. So if bad fruit keeps returning…" I even read verses in the Bible where Jesus explained that it's seemingly *impossible* for good trees to produce bad fruit (see Matthew 7:17-20).

What did that make me?

(In the end, I looked out the attic window and across my backyard. I decided that Jesus must have been speaking in generalities. The best tree at my house occasionally produced a "bad apple." And the most dis-eased tree occasionally exhibited a good one. He looked at the overall trajectory, the thing the tree is known by- not the occasional outlier. As his little brother later wrote in James 3:2, "We all stumble.")

Anyway, the CR leader who gave me the book also directed me to an info table where they kept a dozen or more "green sheets." Each one detailed a specific

---

[35] https://en.wikipedia.org/wiki/Perennial_plant

addiction issue- that is, an incorrect heart attachment. Those pages contained info on everything from *codependency* to *alcoholism* to *having been raised in a dysfunctional family* to *eating disorders* to *mental health issues* to *just about anything else you could brainstorm*. Each sheet listed both symptoms and possible solutions. And every solution required going beneath the surface, heading right into the dirt, and digging deep.

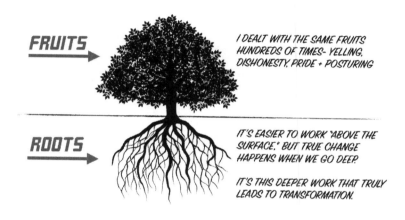

FRUITS → *I DEALT WITH THE SAME FRUITS HUNDREDS OF TIMES- YELLING, DISHONESTY, PRIDE + POSTURING*

ROOTS → *IT'S EASIER TO WORK "ABOVE THE SURFACE," BUT TRUE CHANGE HAPPENS WHEN WE GO DEEP.*

IT'S THIS DEEPER WORK THAT TRULY LEADS TO TRANSFORMATION.

After (just being honest), cussing under my breath, things became ultra-clear to me. **Though most of us never get diagnosed, we all struggle with our demons, it seems. Some of them are just more acceptable, and bit more sanitized, more mainstream, and therefore less noticeable than others.** Though my addictions were acceptable by most standards, they were as equally deadly as their less sanitized counterparts.

I walked out the room, my stack of green sheets in hand, realizing I had a long road ahead of me. By my own estimation, I had 95-100% of the symptoms on several of the "hurts, habits, and hangups" referenced by CR.

But I wasn't afraid. I wasn't afraid if anyone knew. I wasn't afraid that owning the label- even all of the labels- might negate my worth as a person- or even diminish the calling God placed on my life. I'm confident His love is unconditional. And I'm certain His acceptance, His gifts, and His calling are *irrevocable*- even if other people's approval of me is (Romans 11:29).

If He could work around Noah's drunkenness, Abraham's pimping his wife (twice), Jacob's ongoing deception, Moses' anger-management issues, David's adultery, Peter's denials, Paul's murders… then He could certainly work with my "green sheets."

That meant **I just needed to work on my heart- to continue doing the tough work of the soul, the "inside job" of uncovering the facets of the *Imago Dei*, the image of God, that were already tucked inside of me. As I did more of that, more of the fruit I wanted would naturally emerge.**

MISSING THE IMPORTANT

During that long season when I began pulling these ideas together I texted my kids' mom.

"I missed a lot chasing my empty dreams," I typed. "There's nothing- or very little- to show for all of that time away, all of those missed moments, all of those sacrificed seasons…"

In the same way that those addicts have very little to show for all of their addicting behaviors, I had little to show for mine.

"You have no idea," she replied.

The irony is that I forfeited the very relationships which add the most value to my life by chasing things I hoped would fill my life with meaning and purpose.

I remembered something I'd read in my Enneagram book. I reached for the shelf and grabbed it:

> The relationships of spiritually unevolved Threes suffer because they're almost all workaholics. They have so many projects remaining and so many goals to achieve they can't give their undivided attention to people they love.[36]

That was one of my "sins of choice," workaholism. I remembered-

- Always taking work with me on vacation

- Arriving late for dinner- at least 3 or more times each week

- Regularly sending my wife to bed alone while I worked on my computer, pounding away on some project

- Going out with the boys on a Saturday morning sneak out (one of my staples) and slipping into "work mode" as soon as I picked up a book, a blank journal, or a device (it never began that way, but it became another opportunity to put 1-2 hours into something)

Why? Because my heart had been attached to the wrong things.

As *The Road Back to You* says-

> … they all believe in the same lie: you're only as loved as your latest success.[37]

Or, you could flip it: "You're as *unloved* as your latest catastrophe or failure."

---

36 *The Road Back to You*, page 140.

37 See page 142 of *The Road Back to You*.

I had a lot of those failures. And, in large part that's why I covered them. And it's why I rarely asked for help. Admitting I couldn't make something work was akin to confessing that something was wrong with me, that I wasn't worthy of love.

So-

- I cut corners to achieve

- I plowed through people and their feelings in order to chase my dreams

- I hid

- I lied

I was addicted to finding my value, my self-worth, in externals. So, I did the things addicts do. Instead of connecting to the right thing, I connected to the wrong things. Again, **an addiction is *anything* that wrongfully takes the place of primacy in our hearts.**

That night via text, our kids' mom affirmed that she had needed me, that our children *desperately* needed me. That they just wanted to be with their Daddy. That they would go to work with me just to be near me- even when it meant the only time and attention they received was during the car ride back and forth. That they approached me when I left early or came back late because they craved my affirmation.

That's what addiction does. That is, it's what happens when *anything* takes the place of primacy in our hearts- that special spot reserved uniquely for the Creator. Our hearts remain restless until He alone resides there. (*And, even after that, let's be honest, life still feels shaken sometimes, right?*)

AND BACK TO THE THREE FACTS

What does this have to do with emotional pain?

Well, **most of us- because of those 3 Facts and the one about avoiding pain- dodge emotional pain. That is, we're not immune to the things that create the trauma; but we like to avoid *feeling* it.**

So, we cover it. We cling to other things.

We fill the holes that emotional wounds create with things that don't sting, with externals that *feel* good. Money, sex, and drugs... yes. But we also fill that void with things that aren't "sin" issues, things that are actually right and good and even noble.

(*And even sex and money are noble with the right expressions, right?*)

In other words, we dodge doing the tough work of the soul, walking through the dark night until we see the sun, once again rise on our lives. After all, it's much easier to plug a fluorescent into the wall.

So...

- Recent divorcees become "super fit."

- Former addicts take up new hobbies.

- Surviving widows or widowers search for new relationships.

- The abused spouse becomes an advocate and activist.

- Abandoned men and women become workaholics.

I know. Those are all clichés. Seems kind of unfair to pen them like that, because they're stereotypes. The reality is that people come in all shapes and sizes, and we choose our emotional fillers in our own unique ways.

Plus, let's be honest. Some of those activities I just listed are bold, world-changing endeavors. We need more of them. But **we need the those activities we enjoy in conjunction with the deep work of the heart, the hard work of digging the roots and renovating the self from the inside out. Apart from that, they're unhealthy attachments filling a void that can't be filled by an external.**

That's where I had gone. Somewhere along the path, I tethered my heart to the wrong things. Or to the right things in the wrong way.

It was time for me to discover who I really was. To go back to the bottom. To find myself overwhelmed by grace. To rewrite the story. And to let it take as long as it takes- just like I do when I'm writing an actual book.

And that requires, as we'll see in the next chapter, that meant slowing down. Way down.

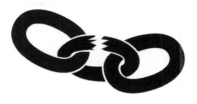

7. The Pause is Often Enough

I wrestled in high school. Though an aggressive sport which pits one man against another in a battle of strength, stamina, and technique, very few accidents and injuries ever occurred during the six years I participated. On the rare instances when they did, wrestling tournaments always stopped. Everything in the entire gym halted. Bouts on other mats paused. Cheerleaders silenced their chants. Conversations in the stands ceased. And- this one's big- most of the competitors *took a knee*, waiting with respect and reverence as we waited for the injured man to arise.

When the wounded athlete, the man in the arena, finally stood to his feet everyone cheered. Even the opponent's team. And people who didn't know the injured man at all.

All because someone was physically hurt…

This leads me to an essential question, a follow-up to the observation: *What if we took a knee for emotional wounds, too?*

PERHAPS STOP A MOMENT

If someone hurts themselves physically, it's not uncommon to take time off from work- or even undergo physical therapy. In fact, we *encourage* them to take their time getting well.

"Recover," we tell them. "Your body needs to rest. You're worth the time it takes to heal."

Looking back, I realize I got this one wrong. A lot. For instance, I *didn't* encourage my wife to take time to emotionally recover after miscarrying a child. I didn't even think about it *either time* it happened. I look back in the rearview mirror and ponder, "What was I thinking?"

Other times I got it right- like the time I suggested we cease extracurricular activities for a season after some trauma in our family came to light... so that we could rally together as a family.

And I *did* have the opportunity to slow down, step back, and deal with my soul issues for about 18 months- but that was because I work from home.

In general, though, **we don't look at people who are emotionally reeling and say, "Hey, take a time out. Let's pause. You need to rest and recover. I'll I'll sit down with you- and not try to fix you- just sit- while you do."**[38]

Over the past year or so it occurred to me that in the same way we encourage someone with a bodily ailment to seek physical therapy (or cheer someone who

---

[38] See Job 2:11f. Everything in his story goes well- as far as the friends are concerned- until they attempt to rationalize the situation and begin pontificating.

says, "Hey, tomorrow I'm going to the gym- I just hired a trainer so I can take control of my health!"), we applaud people who seek other forms of help, as well.

We commend people who take extra classes or go back to school to acquire new knowledge and "shore up" their perceived intellectual / knowledge deficiencies.

We do the exact same thing when someone seeks answers to deeper spiritual questions. We applaud people who set appointments with pastors and spiritual directors.

But what about emotional health? What about internal wounds?

When's the last time you heard someone say, "Hey, I'm taking charge of my emotional health? I'm going to meet with a therapist!", and took them seriously?

If someone said they're going to therapy, would your first thought be, "Wow! Courageous! Do the tough work of the soul!"… or would it be, "Hmmm… I wonder's what's wrong with them?" instead?

WOUNDED HEARTS

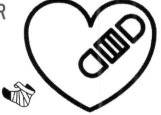

WHAT IF WE CARED FOR WOUNDED EMOTIONS LIKE WE CARE FOR WOUNDED BODIES?

For years I wanted to run from emotions rather than running towards them. It seemed safer, easier. Yet the way towards health and healing is actually to move straight into the emotions rather than trying to navigate around them. The truth is that "without a healthy physical heart, your body cannot survive, and life ceases to exist. The same is true for this metaphysical heart."[39]

You see, **pain isn't the enemy emotionally anymore than it is physically.** Most of us do our best to avoid emotional pain. We bury it. We explain it away.

Think about the need for pain, though...

PAIN IS NOT YOUR ENEMY

A few years ago, my son Judah broke his arm. He tripped on the playground, landed awkwardly as he tried to catch himself, and snapped his forearm in half. Every kid and teacher on the playground actually *heard* it.

The break was so thorough that he had to hold the "broken" part of his arm in place lest it just dangle. I gently tied his arm to his body with some cut-up cloths and rushed him to the doctor. The physical wound was *obvious*.

About a year later my daughter Mini fell from the zip line in our backyard.[40] She was shaken up a bit, so we took her inside and let her take a warm bath.

An hour or two post-fall, she complained of pain in her wrist. It looked fine- no dangling loose like Judah's left arm- but the pain persisted. So, I loaded her in the car with one of her older sisters who had broken an arm before for moral support.

---

39 Christa Black Smith, *Heart Made Whole*, Kindle version- location 302.

40 Her real name is Miriam. Mini is my nickname. It's a story for another time.

We took her to the emergency room and learned she had a small sprain- all because of the pain.

Or, to say it another way, her wound wasn't obvious like Judah's. *If she didn't experience the pain we wouldn't have known about the sprain.*

In the same way physical pain alerts us to the notion that something isn't quite right in our bodies, emotional pain reveals the truth about our souls. Emotional wounds tell us that something's not quite right. We actually *need* the pain.

But, remember, we like to avoid pain (*Fact 2*), so it's easy to cover this one up and keep going...

Think about it.

I mean, pause and really think about it.

And think about what *might* happen if we took emotional healing seriously. If we...

- *Encouraged emotional exploration and growth like we foster intellectual endeavors?*

- *Treated emotional hurts with the same care we use for spiritual questions?*

- *Explored what's happening inside of us before we tried to connect relationally with those around us, propping on them to bandaid our feelings before we even understand what's there?*

- *Paused and took the necessary time to deal with the emotional traumas like we do for physical wounds?*

If you've followed my website or my podcast for any length of time, you know that I'm a proponent of Divine healing. Yes, I'll visit a medical doctor if we need to (as I did for both Judah and Mini)- so I'm definitely not anti-medical (even though we prefer natural health options)- but if something major happens we're also praying.[41] Many times we see physical miracles.

I'll be honest with you. When I went to church services and people said something like, "Yeah, we saw a few people emotionally healed," I used to think it was a cop out. I valued physical healing more- *because it was quantifiable.* You could see it. The results were *measurable.*

I've learned I was short-sighted in overlooking emotional health + healing.

DIFFERENT PEOPLE = DIFFERENT PAIN TOLERANCE

I shared all of this at the dinner table with a few friends one night. As we pondered the reality that we often applaud all other types of healing and advancement except emotional healing- and tend to just push through when we face emotional hurts- I listened to a State Trooper, a U.S. vet from the Iraq War, and a first responder discuss their past traumas with me.

"Having people shoot at me in Iraq was nothing," the vet said. "I mean, I've heard stories- and know guys- who suffered from PTSD because our unit got mortared so

---

41 Example: Judah and Mini both went to the doctor in the previous two examples.

many times. That didn't phase me. The thing that set me back the most was getting sexually abused when I was a little boy."

The first responder went next: "I've had my life threatened, too. But the biggest trauma I faced was when the guy who trained me was killed in the line of duty. It was my day off when it happened, so I wasn't there with him. I felt guilty about it for years. Sometimes I still do. That really messed me up, even though I wasn't there to experience it. Maybe there's something I could have done. I should have been there. I wonder about it a lot."

The State Trooper told us, "They always train troopers with a seasoned leader. Before they send us on our own in a patrol car they want us to work at least one fatality on the highway…" He continued, "Coming up on the scene like that is hard, because you never know what to expect. It can take hours to sort through everything, get the accident cleared, and do everything you have to do. Then, after you've worked it you have to drive to the family member's house and let them know. To me, letting someone I didn't even know that someone else I didn't even know died a horrific, unexpected death was the worst. I'm not sure why it affected me like it did."

From these men I put together one common theme about emotional pain: **Emotional pain rattles us, yet we all tend to under-value it once we realize where the wound originated.** Each of these guys realized there were issues in the lives which could have been perceived as "bigger deals." Rightfully so. Each one admitted there were "bigger" things that caused issues for others. That is, someone else always has it "worse off."

We all perceive trauma differently. The things which prove hard for me may seem easy to you. And the situation that may send you into emotional upheaval might hardly register on my pain scale at all.

Emotional hurts and pains are unique to each person. So, rather than undermining how we feel when something heartfelt occurs (whether we caused it or not, whether it's the result of our own sin or a sin committed against us), we should simply deal with it the best we can where we are.

Compare it to physical injuries for a moment:

- Three of Mini's four brothers fell from that same zip line at different times, simply dusted the grass off their clothes, and zipped again.

- Over the years, hundreds of kids have fell on the playground where Judah tripped and *never* broke their arms.

- Thousands of takedowns happened at those wrestling tournaments with no incident at all.

People respond to physical pain differently. It only makes sense that we would respond to emotional pains differently as well.

That means *only you* can communicate how something affected you. In other words, you must confront the pain in order to heal it, because *you* are the pain scale.

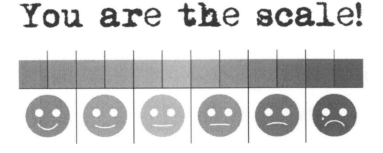

THE PAUSE IS SOMETIMES ENOUGH

Let me take you back to the wrestling mat for a moment and share with you something I remember as I was putting this chapter together. It's so common that you've probably seen it before.

Whether he could continue the bout or not, as the wounded athlete stood to his feet, the crowds *always* cheered. It didn't matter who we were cheering for before the injury. After waiting to see what happened, *we all celebrated for him.*

And, there's this...

Most of the time, after resting for a few minutes and catching his breath, the injured athlete was able to actually continue the match. Fighting with a renewed vigor- and with scores of people now in his corner- he often finished the mat with his hand raised. That is, he triumphed. **Don't miss the fact that sometimes the simple pause was enough. It enabled the man to catch his breath, to gather his wits, and to face the battle courageously and victoriously.**

I believe it's the same way with emotional hurts and pains, too. Often, living an intentional rhythm of Sabbath and sleep provides sacred space, deliberate pauses, where the mess of life gets sorted and we're able to not only stand but also step back to the center of the mat.

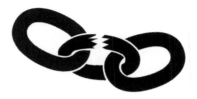

8. Five Signs You're Out of Rhythm

About a decade ago I made the swap from Windows-based computers to Apple. The upside is that all of my devices connect and communicate with one another seamlessly. If I type something into the Notes app on my iPhone, it appears on my laptop. And if I edit it *there*, the corrections automatically appear- almost magically- on the desktop in my home office. This interconnectivity skyrocketed my productivity and the ease with which I navigate my workflow.

Again, that's the upside.

Yes, there's also a downside. It's a tricky one, but it's there. Here's my shot explaining it…

Apple products just, well, they just *work*. It seems like the other kinds of computers I used were always finicky and regularly flat-lined. They took forever to start-up. Every time a program got "locked up" I had to reboot the entire machine. The "blue screen of death" regularly appeared. I had to purchase a new computer- almost like precision clockwork- every year. And, since nothing transferred automatically (I spent numerous sleepless nights struggling in vain to sync, move, clone, etc.), I had to reinstall every program individually and adjust every setting on the new computer. I've never had to do any of that with my Macs.

I know. You're wondering, "What's the downside?"

Turns out, my Mac laptops have worked so well that I never even turn them off. Ever. I just press "Control + S" (the macro to save the current file) and then close the cover. That's it.

When I want to work again, I just open the computer like a book and begin anew-any changes I pecked into my phone or any other device having already *automatically* made their way to the never-turned-off-laptop.

Yet there's the rub.

Eventually, my first Mac began dragging. Struggling. Bad. It began behaving like a Windows-based PC. The whole thing got janky enough that I set an appointment at the Genius Bar at the local Apple Store.

"Do you ever turn this thing off?" the blue-shirted Genius asked me.

Knowing I was probably "in trouble" by a kid half my age, I sheepishly admitted, "Uh... no. Not really." Then, after a few moments, "Actually, not at all."

"Let's restart it," he said.

He punched a few keys and did something I hadn't done to the computer in 6-9 months: *he powered the machine down.* Completely off.

After a few minutes, he pressed the power button and the laptop came back to life-almost as if it was completely new. Over the next few days, I noticed that the computer no longer slogged along. It's like the entire system exhibited renewed vigor and enthusiasm.

Crazy, huh?

If you've own a cell phone (I know, the technical name is *mobile* phone, now, and everybody has one), you've probably had unresolvable issues with it, called tech support, and then heard them tell you something like, "Alright, do this for me. Let's perform something called a *hard reset*. We're going to completely power the thing down, wait a few moments, and then start it back up."

They always promise something that seems absurd for such a simple task as turning the phone off: "That should fix it."

Generally, they're right. It does.

I've seen this with virtually all of my electronic devices. I have a huge 55" TV in my living room. Tied to my Apple TV, I leave it on all the time. I play music from it and let the screen-saver run in the background… 24 hours a day.

About once a week, though, the sound just stops working. Everything goes *silent*.

It flustered me the first time I discovered this phenomena. I sat down, pizza in hand, ready to enjoy a movie at the end of a long week of work-travel with my compadres Jim Bob & Ernie. I left the television "on" the entire time we were gone, of course.

Imagine my un-delight when I selected a movie from my Wish List, settled back to enjoy, and watched the opening bumper begin to play… *in complete silence*. I decided if the *power-off-WAIT-power-on* routine was good enough for the tiny phone it was probably good enough for the sound function of my over-sized TV.

Worked like a charm.

Now, without fail, the occasional quiet spell phases-me-not. I take it in stride. I power everything off, pause, re-power it, and everything *instantly* works again. Like new. **The temporary pause creates space where the machine performs at max output once again.**

I restart my computer at least once a week, now. And I regularly turn the phone completely off. When I do, they work well. When I don't, they just *don't*. Until I do a hard reset, that is.

Notice the graphic below. **The more trips I make around the sun the more I realize we're exactly like those machines. In order to "work right" we've got to pause, too**.

WHAT DO THESE HAVE IN COMMON?

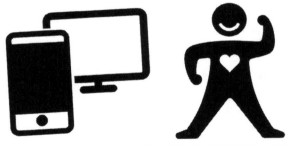

EACH NEEDS A REGULAR "HARD RESET" TO FUNCTION PROPERLY!

A few months ago we released the book *Healthy Hustle*.[42] I titled chapter 1 "Creation's Rhythm," the main argument being that for all the talk in our culture

---

[42] https://www.oilyapp.com/HealthyHustle for more info. Or, go to www.OilyApp.com/books for ordering info.

about living in balance, that's not how we're designed to live. **We're made-we're hardwired-** *not to live in balance but to live in rhythm.* That is, we're created to live in segments of high intensity followed by breaks of complete rest.

Power on. Power off. Power on. Power off. Power on. Power off...

That's not how we usually run things, though. In fact, when we face tough situations we may actually tend to grind away faster and harder, thinking that more effort will help us "fix it," whatever it is...

Rather than making forward progress, though, the result is often like trying to drive a stuck truck out the mud. **The harder you push, the "more stuck" you become. In fact, fairly fast you realize the weight you're carrying and the energy you're expending actually work** *against* **you.** You regress rather than progress...

At some point, in order to unstick a truck you've got to *pause.* You've got to step out and knock off some of the mud. That is, **you've got to be willing to** *not* **make progress for a moment in order to actually meaningfully progress at all...**

Now think about that- *and how it applies to life.* And to the hurts and wounds we carry from the hard things we've endured. The best way to move forward is (like the computer, the phone, and the truck) to live in rhythm. In fact, that's the best way to get to wholeness when we're broken, and it's the best way to remain there once we make it.

So how can you tell if you're living in rhythm?

Sometimes, it's easier to see something based on what it *doesn't* look like. After all, if we're living out of sync, we probably resemble the symptoms of living off-beat rather than living on.

For the remainder of this chapter, I'll outline five signs that you might be out of sync. Here they are-

1. You can't get quiet, don't want to be alone, etc.

2. You often feel sickish or sluggish for no reason

3. You're snappy

4. You feel down or depressed

5. You've just endured trauma or hard things

As we discuss them, I'll provide you with some tips to move back to the cadence for which you were created.

ONE = YOU CAN'T GET QUIET, DON'T WANT TO BE ALONE, ETC.

One of the essential oil blends in Young Living's Freedom Sleep kit is Valor, an oil usually associated with "facing hard things." The name is a nod to the Roman soldiers who are said to have placed a similar blend of oils on the soles of their feet and on their shields before marching into battle. Courage, a synonym of Valor, doesn't deny fear. Rather, it acknowledges the tension of continuing amidst it, anyway. Just like those ancient warriors.

As we met to shoot a video course about the kit, I asked Jim Bob, "Why is Valor in the Sleep kit? Wouldn't that make more sense in the Freedom Release kit? The Sleep kit is for going to bed. The Release it is for facing the day…"[43]

"Well, it's true that the Sleep kit is more for pausing to rest and recover and then the Release kit is more for living whole, but sometimes the most courageous thing people can do is to actually stop and pause," JB said. Then- **"Think about how many things people do to occupy themselves in order to avoid being quiet, still, or alone."**

I thought about what he said for a moment. And I thought back to my recent "history" with my phone.

Then I looked down at my mobile phone. It was on. For the most part, it stays on. Even when I sleep, the phone is on.

I thought about the weekly report Apple sends me, detailing how much time I spent on the phone each day- on average. They also outline which apps were the biggest culprits.

"5.5 hours," one report said.

I looked at it. Closely. That was almost 6 hours *per day* that my screen was on with my eyeballs facing it!

Yes, I churn a lot of my work on social media, *but not that much*. I generally create my graphics and write my copy on my computer, then- since my Apple devices sync- I let the content "cross-over" to the phone *on its own*. Through "the cloud." I copy and paste the images and text from there. That means that 5.5 hours didn't

---

[43] Watch the course at www.OilyApp.com/Freedom.

include any of my screen time on the laptop, which is the place I actually spent the majority of my "device time."

In fact, here's just how much time I spend on the laptop- in addition to that 5.5 hours…

Over the past 12 months- as of typing this page you're currently reading- I wrote in excess of 2,000 pages of content. I produced 7 video courses. I created several hundred graphics for social media. Yes, that's my "job," but however you slice it, that makes the 5.5 hours of screen time on the phone a bit absurd- because, again, it's all an *add-on* to the laptop. And that's an *add-on* to the desktop I use to edit our videos.

I decided to knock the screen time down. The phone part. Since I don't mindlessly surf the Internet from my laptop, only opening it when I'm sitting to actually work, the phone is my culprit.

I cut the time. Quickly. I seriously contemplated removing the apps and turning my smartphone into a "dumb phone," only deciding not to do so because I would need to grab another phone or an iPad (yet *another* screen) in order to handle my social media feeds. In the end, it was just easier to do the phone the right way rather than create a series of workarounds.

All those thoughts about the phone rambling in my mind, I looked back at JB. Remember, we were talking about why Valor was in the Sleep kit rather than the Release kit. I shrugged my shoulders. Like the "whatever" emoji in the phone.

"I think you're right," I told him. "The last 18 months was the hardest season of my life. During that time I wrote more pages than I imagined possible and I concurrently watched more Netflix series- every show in the entire series- than I can count. I spent a lot of time alone, doing the hard work of the soul, but that was intentional. It would have been easier to turn the TV back on and just stay on my white futon for a few hours…"

"A lot of people are like that," he said. "That's why people scroll Facebook while they're laying in the bed at night…"

"And," I replied, half-way confessing, "why they hit Instagram first thing in the morning, before they roll out of bed…"

"Yep," JB continued. "And it's why they look at their social feeds while sitting at the traffic lights when they're driving."

"We've lost the ability to just be bored, to just be quiet. To just be alone."

Then, "Does anybody even sit *on the toilet* anymore without looking at a phone?"

Good question, right?

I thought about all the alone-time I spent over the past 18 months. Sometimes *that* was harder than any other thing. That quiet space became the tough place.

I continued, "I understand why Valor is in the Sleep kit, now. **The bravest thing some people can do- the most courageous or valiant activity- is to actually stop. Pause. Confront the whispers they hear in the silence.**"

I read Michael Hyatt's book *Free to Focus* this past year. He writes about doing "less" stuff so that you can really zero-in on what you want to do. Then, he discusses the importance of margin, of living with quiet space. That is, do less stuff. And do it less of the time.

Hyatt tells of a phrase he and his wife learned while traveling through Tuscany while on a sabbatical (he unplugs for an entire month every summer), *a dolce far niente.* It means "the sweetness of doing nothing." That is, it's not only a refusal to fill every space with *something*, it's a celebration of that space where *nothing else* exists.

Hyatt reminds us,

> *Our brains aren't designed to run nonstop. When we drop things into neutral, ideas flow on their own, memories sort themselves out, and we give ourselves a chance to rest.*[44]

And,

> *Sufficient sleep keeps us mentally sharp and improves our ability to remember, learn, and grow. It refreshes our emotional state, reduces stress, and recharges our bodies... Meanwhile, going without sleep makes it harder to stay focused, solve problems, make good decisions, or even play with others.*[45]

To summarize in my own words, "**The quiet space is where the magic happens**."

Turns out, we don't have any space for magic. We fill it with smartphones + film series + memes + sound-bites + anything else which can hold out attention. **We don't value the pause; we value productivity**. And that productivity- whether it's notching off another project or checking off another social feed or film- often masks the fact that we're afraid to confront that quiet. To borrow language we used in a previous chapter, **sometimes we're addicted to the noise.**

Are you nervous about getting quiet, hitting the pause button, and spending a bit of time on your own in silence...?

That might be a sign you're living out of rhythm.

---

[44] See Michael Hyatt's *Free to Focus*, pp36-37.

[45] Michael Hyatt, *Free to Focus*, p70.

TWO = YOU OFTEN FEEL SICKISH OR SLUGGISH FOR NO REASON

When I ran Windows-based computers, it seems like I got a new "Trojan Horse" virus every few weeks. Hidden in email attachments, located in enticing webforms, or buried in software downloads, those pleasant-looking files carried hidden cargo-small warriors waiting to unleash their fury on the hard drive. When they did, the entire system began to drag. The boondoggle was so culturally pervasive that entire companies like McAfee and Norton ballooned overnight by selling somewhat workable solutions to the fiasco.

(It still baffles me that my Mac runs virtually virus-free.)

Now, think of your body like a computer *again*. In the same way you need a regular reset in order to keep performing, when something goes amok internally, your entire "hard drive" gets sluggish. Most people understand this on a physical level. An upset stomach, a small infection, or a headache can toss your entire body half-speed. **Many people don't realize, though, that the same thing is true emotionally, mentally, and even spiritually. When one area gets affected, they're all affected**.

The solution for ridding your computer of a virus is to download the correct software and then to… you probably guessed it… *reboot the entire system*. That's right, *turn it off*.

It almost sounds too simple, doesn't it?

Yet we don't do it with our computers because we don't want the "down time" from work. We can't pause the output. So, we endure with shoddy operating systems.

The same thing happens in "real life." *To us.* We don't want to slow down. We're *too busy* to slow down.

Remember Michael Hyatt's lines from a few pages ago, though. **Sleep is when your body rebuilds and when your mind goes to rest and begins processing and mending and "figuring out" the stuff from your day. It's when you reset- *completely*. It's when you *heal*.**

Oddly enough, this is such a massive concept that even business books are being written- not about mission or vision or the other things we typically attribute to biz- about getting more sleep. And naps.

There are 5 stages of sleep. Most people never get out of that first bit where you're halfway asleep, halfway awake. That place where dreams and real life blur. That place where you "dream" an intruder is breaking into your home, but it's just a kid walking into your room and tapping you on the shoulder. That place where you continue waking up confused about what's real and what's the dream.

When you don't get enough rest, it flips your body's internal cadence upside down and backwards. You begin running on adrenalin at night (such that you can't sleep) and you begin crashing during the day (you constantly yawn, always need coffee, and desperately crave a nap).

You *look* Zombie-like.

(Your close friends might even mention it!)

You *feel* sluggish and sickish.

Remember, too, that your body needs rest when it's awake, too- space when you're not looking at your phone, occupying every minute. Your mind craves the quiet- even if your thoughts initially rebel against it.

When's the last time you day-dreamed?

Turns out, day-dreaming works a lot like sleep. It's a time when your mind wanders, makes the connections you need, and begins creatively processing hidden data in your hard drive. The majority of my best ideas spontaneously emerge *from nothing* when I'm not thinking about anything except the exercise I'm enjoying in the moment...

In her book *Grunt*, Mary Roach recounts her lessons from the military.[46] She says they studied soldiers who lacked sleep and discovered when we get less than 8 hours a night for 2 weeks in a row, we begin operating at the same diminished capacity we would if we had too much to drink. Except we haven't. And it's going on all day, every day. It's like a perpetual hang-over.

Do you feel sluggish or sickish for no legitimate reason?

Think about it. It could be a sign you're out of rhythm.

THREE = YOU'RE SNAPPY

I have seven biological kids. At various seasons, I've had even more in my home. Each one has their unique personality, their own quirks, and the traits that make them uniquely themselves- even though they've all been raised in the exact same environment.

Here's one thing they all have in common, though: *when they were little and got too tired, they all morphed into midget minions.*

---

[46] *Grunt*, Mary Roach, https://amzn.to/2VuT0gj.

They got snappy. They fought over toys (even the ones they weren't even playing with). They couldn't complete their sentences. They became tyrant-toddlers.

No kidding.

My kids were (they still are) incredible. They were obedient, tender, and looked out for each other. They generally believed the best in others and played.

Unless tired. If they got too tired, all bets were off.

Then, I knew it was time to just say something like, "Hey, you're manifesting something that's not quite you... let's go lay down and start over in an hour or so."

Or, if it was late in the day, "Let's go brush your teeth and hit the B-E-D. You don't even have to take a bath tonight. You've had a long one. Tomorrow is a new day."

The results were predictably awesome. Every time, the kid awakened as if resurrecting from the dead. Their manners returned, their kindness was back, they were brand new little people. **Turns out, they weren't emotionally devastated- even though they acted like it. They were just tired.**

Now, apply this *to you*.

If you're having trouble sorting through some clutter, getting along with others, or find yourself overwhelmed with a situation, it may be that you just need more sleep. In the same way toddlers get (legit) crazy and we recognize that they just need a bit of rest so that they can handle reality, adults are the same way.

Are you snappy? Cranky? Like an over-sized toddler a wee bit too much of the time?

It could be a sign... you might be out of rhythm.

FOUR = YOU FEEL DEPRESSED AND CAN'T FIGURE OUT WHY

Last Fall I found myself sitting in a nearby coffee shop. (I find myself in places like that a lot.) As I finished typing a chapter for a project I was completing, I stared out the oversized storefront window next to my table. Outside, the day was *perfect*. It *wasn't* one of those dreary, grey-colored days that makes you feel foggy.

Yet, as a closed the computer (without turning it off, of course), I thought, "I'm *really* tired."

Inside, something was brewing. Something wasn't quite right…

I looked back outside. Sometimes the weather makes me feel tired, as if my body mimics what happens in the environment. Clearly, this *wasn't* that, though.

"Why am I tired?" I pondered. "I went to bed last night around 8pm, watched a movie, and then slept 10 full hours. This doesn't make sense…"

Then I thought about the bigger life situation in which I found myself. I looked at my phone (always on, *right?*) and re-read the previous few text messages. A once-close companion had drawn a sword against me. I realized I wasn't tired as I sat there in the coffee shop, *I was depressed…*

And, no, I might not have met the clinical definition such that a professional could diagnose, treat, and prescribe me, but I was clearly down…

Now, get this, depression and tiredness often mirror each other. In other words-

- Depression can make you feel tired

- Being tired can make you feel like your depressed

Sometimes, you're both. Other times, **your soul (depressed) dictates to your body how it should feel (tired). Then, there are times when your body (tired) makes your soul feel something that might not actually be (depressed)**.

That day at the coffee shop, *I was depressed*. Clearly. If I told you the story- the one happening in real life at that moment (and not just one playing in my head) you'd probably agree, "Yeah, I can see why you would be depressed. And I understand why that would make you feel really, really tired."

I've learned a few things about myself through experience.

- Sometimes, when I feel a little down (especially now that I'm not afraid of words like *depression* nor fearful of confronting the fact that I might feel *blue*) I can actually recognize when I'm just physically exhausted- so tired that my body's need for rest brings my entire soul down with it, as if begging me to give myself a break.

- At other times when I can't separate the two and tell which one is which, I've learned I can eliminate the variables by taking a break. I ease back from the computer and go for a stroll around the block, coffee in hand. Or I take a brisk run. If it's late, I just go to bed.

When I know that I'm not being lazy, that I'm stewarding my time well and proactively doing the work the Lord has granted me to do with diligence, I can confidently take a solid pause when my body tells me I need it. Then, the feelings tend to buff.

Do you ever feel depressed?

You might be. Or you might just be tired. Either way, it might be a sign that you need to step back into rhythm.

FIVE = YOU'VE JUST ENDURED TRAUMA OR HARD THINGS

Most people can't- and shouldn't- make major decisions in the midst of trauma or when they're unusually tired. **When you're in the middle of something hard, the best thing you can do is step back, catch your breathe, and wait. Very rarely will you make things worse by waiting**. Rushing, on the other hand, creates all kinds of chaos.

(Also, most truly golden opportunities aren't "now or never," regardless of the story we tell ourselves.)

Let me explain via a story…

A few years ago an elder in our church lost in his mother-in-law in a tragic car accident. I was studying at a coffee shop when I received the phone call. Oddly enough, several of the elders and staff members from our church planned to eat dinner at his house that evening. Unmarried, the MIL had been on the way to purchase groceries *for us*.

This happened on a Saturday. The next week, we all paused *everything* while we helped him and his wife sort their "new normal." A few of us joined his wife at the funeral home to navigate caskets and costs and decisions which had to be made for burial. Others kept kids. Others set up meal trains or ran family errands.

I drew three *other* straws.

First, I accompanied my friend to visit family members and tell them the news. That is, I delivered the "death notices" with him. Due to where he was emotionally, I did most of the talking. It was surreal and raw, as many of the extended family members denied the reality we tenderly delivered to them and expressed completely predictable reactions to hearing tough news.

Second, I rode to the tow truck lot to gather personal effects and remove other belongings from the totaled SUV. His wife didn't want to see the vehicle in which her mother, who had been her best friend, was killed. Understandably, he didn't want to go alone. I climbed into the half-crushed car and retrieved several items.

Third, I drove my friend to the law firm where his MIL worked as a paralegal for a big-name attorney in town. Same thing. We needed to gather her belongings like people do when they retire and move out for good. He didn't want to handle the errand, moving her out of her office ten years too early, by himself.

Looking back at each of these three snapshots, there's no way he could have made the trek by himself. He had just been T-boned with some of the worse news you can ever hear. There was no prep period for it; it was totally unexpected. It made sense that he needed someone to literally tell him where to go, what to say, and when it was time to leave and move to the next item on his growing list of things to handle postmortem.

While we were at the attorney's office, he discovered he needed to handle one more thing. And he didn't want to be there alone for it either- even though it was intensely personal. We needed to resolve her life insurance policy. The firm provided one to care for her family in the event of an unlikely death. In that moment, we stood in the midst of the *unlikely event* no one thought would ever happen.

"I need you there," he told me. "I don't know that I'll be to remember anything they say, and I've never done this before."

I was honored to go, to be trusted to help him meander through such horrible moments.

We sat in the office, thinking we were about to receive a check for about $10,000- slightly more than the burial expenses. However, the gracious boss before us explained that he and his wife (also a partner at the firm) adored the MIL and her family, and that they increased the original policy on her behalf to provide the same coverage as the partners at the firm received.

"She meant the world to us," he said. "You never think anything like this will happen, but we wanted to make sure her family was cared for if it ever did." He reached across the mahogany desk that all attorneys use and handed my friend a check for *multiple 6-figures.*

As the boss left the room, my friend looked at me. Then, "What do I do with this? I wasn't expecting it?"

In that moment, I knew he was looking for leadership- for someone to tell him *exactly* what he should do.

Why?

Because he found himself in the middle of trauma. And **when unresolved emotions are involved, it's almost always impossible to see the path forward**.

I made a list.

I told him slowly and definitively, "I know you have been looking at minivans and have planned to purchase one for your wife and kids for a few months now. Next week, after the funeral is over and the out-of-town guests have gone home, go pay cash for the van like you already planned to do."

"That sounds good," he said. "Then what?"

"Take the rest of this money and put it all in an interest-bearing account for at least one year."

He started taking notes, writing the instructions I offered him.

I continued, "Don't touch the money for a year. None of it. You don't need to make an emotional decision about it. That means not to tithe any of it to our church, not to go do something emotionally-charged in the moment like take everyone in the extended family on a vacation... just let it sit. You weren't expecting it. You don't need it to pay your bills. Time will give you perspective on how to make the most of what she's left you and your family."

Then, after a few moments, I added, "And don't tell *anyone* about this money except for your wife. People will come out of the woodwork wanting money if they know you have it. Keep it quiet."

I also suggested he run my advice by the other three guys who ran the church with us (and their wives), those elders who had been picking up the slack since the car accident. But that was it. Vault it. For at least 365 days.

A year later- almost to the date- my friend approached me after church one Sunday morning.

"We just dropped a check in the offering," he said. "It was from that insurance settlement. Thank you for telling me to wait to do anything with the money. You were right."

As his wife pulled up outside in the white van she'd been driving for the past 11 months or so, he continued, "We would have made so many bad decisions in the moment if we didn't have someone looking in from outside the situation telling me that it was OK- and even best- to just pause for a while. Getting some distance between us and the accident helped bring some perspective. Thank you."

"You would have done the same thing," I offered. "**When you're in crisis, the best thing to do is to let someone you trust help guide you. It's hard to make a decision in those moments. It's best if you can just recover and lean on someone else for a little while.**"

As I mentioned earlier, I worked in drug rehabs, homeless shelters, and prison reentry programs for about about 8 years. Everyday I encountered people in crisis. This one was fleeing an abusive situation. That one was facing court. The other one was staring down legal ramifications that finally caught up with them...

These people were *all* in some form of crisis.

I learned I'm actually skilled at making wise decisions amidst crisis. I don't freeze. I don't fight. I don't get frightened. I can see it all, as if in slow motion- even though you have to sometimes make quick decisions. And, I provide sound counsel that always benefits the other person.

Unless it's my own crisis, that is. Then, since I'm personally involved and invested in the outcome, it's hard for me to navigate. I'm too emotionally charged. At that point, I need to pause and let someone else steer me.

Like most people, I can't make good decisions when I'm tired or knee deep in trauma. So, unless forced to, I don't even try. I step back. I pause. I gather perspective.

Have you been through a traumatic experience lately?

That's hard work. And it's hard to rest and reset while you're in the middle of it. For your long-term health + wholeness, it's worth stepping back and making sure you move into rhythm.

REST FIRST

Young Living has two kits related to emotional hurts and wounds... for invisible scars. The Freedom Sleep kit and the Freedom Release kit work together.

Somehow, in my mind, I mentally placed the Release kit first. But that's not the way they work. It's not the way we're designed to work. Young Living suggests you use the Sleep kit for 30 days, followed by the Release kit for 30 days.

Here's why...

In the *Healthy Hustle* book I wrote about the way in which the ancient Hebrews viewed a 24-hour day. They began their days at sunset, not sunrise. That is, they began with the evening- with rest. That's why we see the refrain through that Genesis 1 that "there was evening and then morning, the _____ day."

The kits acknowledge that **the rhythm of Creation is *rest* first- then *work*. It's the cadence that's true for all of life- particularly for doing the hard work of handling emotional hurts.**

Rather than minimizing our hurts (something we tend to do) and then pushing forward, we acknowledge them. We slow down. We rest, allowing whatever needs to surface to make it's way up- free from the clutter that pushes it down. We recharge. We may find we're still wounded, but at that point we're able to move forward.

Now, pause.

Reflect on what you've just learned about emotional freedom, those five signs that you might be out of rhythm:

1. You can't get quiet, don't want to be alone, etc.

2. You often feel sickish or sluggish for no reason

3. You're snappy

4. You feel down or depressed

5. You've just endured trauma or hard things

Remember, like we saw with the wounded wrestler, many times a simple un-rushed pause is enough to provide the grace and space you need to recuperate and then continue.

When you're ready, turn the page. In the following chapter I'm going to tell you about something that's more powerful than PTSD yet, at the same time, has an uncommonly simple cure.

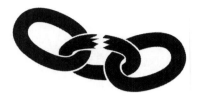

9. More Powerful Than PTSD

Throughout this book we've addressed soul wounds that are primarily mental (our mindset) or emotional (our feelings). But, there's another area we haven't spoken about- namely, spiritual health (our faith).

In the same way our emotions can be "broken," so also can the unique connection between our soul and our spirit. Perhaps this story will help illustrate what I mean...

Washington Booker III is one of the warriors featured in the documentary *Honoring the Code*.[47] I'll explain more about that documentary in a moment.

Booker was a U.S. Marine Corps sniper during the Vietnam War. When he was interviewed for the film, he said bootcamp actually altered his definition of what it meant to be human. At least, it did *for a moment*.

---

[47] Access the film free at www.WarriorHope.com/HTC.

He said, "When you show up for boot camp, and you go to infantry training school, they constantly drill into you that your job is to close in and kill the enemy."

He reminded us there's a tension you feel, because "When you begin, killing is not normal to you. They turn it into something else and make it acceptable. They run you until you almost fall out, and then you yourself begin saying, *Kill! Kill! Kill!* You begin to cheer for something you were once adamantly against."[48]

More relevant to our discussion about overall wholeness, Booker told a story from the battlefield. He reported, "I was a sniper. During a battle I killed an NVA lieutenant.[49] It was about 4 or 5 o'clock in the morning when they hit us. I remembered where he fell..."

Notice what he said. In the same way a hunter makes a mental note as to where the deer or bird fell so that he can later collect it, Booker marked where his target died.

He confessed why: "So I could go and search the body for souvenirs after the battle."

The battle raged most of the day. Late in the afternoon, well after the U.S. forces pushed the Viet Cong troops back, Booker looped back to check the body.

"I checked his belt, and I took his weapon," he said. "Then, I opened his wallet."

Remembering what he saw next, he reminisced, "There were some pictures in there- probably some place in North Vietnam. And in those pictures were him, a woman, and some children. I knew then that they were his wife and his kids."

---

48 Notice that he speaks about a "new normal" here. Often, when emotional wounds happen, they create a new normal for us. We *expect* abuse, trauma, etc.- this changes our perception of reality, like we discussed earlier in the book.

49 NVA = North Vietnamese Army

Those few seconds *changed* him. At bootcamp killing became acceptable. And encouraged. It no longer felt that way. The pendulum jerked back in the opposite direction. An invisible wave of regret crashed over him, submerging him amidst his thoughts as he stood on the battlefield.

Booker revealed, "That very second, the man I killed became a *human*– not a combatant. He was no longer some evil force moving along ridge lines or shadows. He became a *person*. His wife and his kid were now somewhere crying. Needless to say, I never searched another body."

THE UNEXPECTED PLOT TWIST

If you follow me on social media, you know I wrote a book and have created a course for veterans who struggle with the invisible scars of war.[50] I did so in partnership with a nonprofit known as Crosswinds. That's how I got introduced to Booker and his story.

My friend Bob Waldrep founded the organization over a decade ago. Shortly thereafter, as an overflow of some the projects he found himself and his new organization involved in, he launched Front Porch Media & Entertainment in 2012. His goal was to better utilize film as a means of serving others.

It became apparent that the first full-length feature needed to focus on the facet of his organization that focused on public policy and military service, specifically by creating a documentary aimed at helping military personnel who were suffering

---

[50] *Warrior Hope* is the book. Go to WarriorHope.com for more info.

mental and emotional trauma (such as PTSD) as a result of their deployment, combat experience, or separation from family members who had been deployed.

The nonprofit released the first film, *Invisible Scars*, in 2014 and immediately gained wide grassroots distribution- largely by word of mouth. DVDs of the film were passed from person to person, and- through generous donors- provided free to veterans and their families. 40,000 were given away in the first few years. This "accidental" method of mass distribution created a relational connection between the organization, government agencies, service providers, and current and former soldiers.[51]

Here's where it gets super-interesting...

When you film a documentary, you have an idea of where the film will most likely take you, but you've got to remain open to the possibilities that it might take a turn you don't expect. It could lead you somewhere else completely.

Icarus, the documentary which won an Academy Award for Best Documentary Feature, is a prime example. I streamed the film on Netflix one evening and was shocked at the radical turn it took.

The film began as a study in illegal sports doping.[52] The filmmaker wanted to know if he could improve *his* performance with drugs. Along the way, the he connected with a Russian scientist who became a trusted friend, a friend who later revealed

---

[51] Stream the film free at www.InvisibleScars.online.

[52] See https://en.wikipedia.org/wiki/Icarus_(2017_film) for more info. Wiki reports, "While investigating the furtive world of illegal doping in sports, Bryan Fogel connects with Russian scientist, Dr. Grigory Rodchenkov, the director of Russia's national anti-doping laboratory. Rodchenkov creates a plan for Fogel to take banned performance-enhancing drugs in a way that will evade detection from drug-testing, helping Fogel's experiment to prove that the current way athletes are tested for drugs is insufficient. As Fogel continues his training, he and Rodchenkov become friends, and Rodchenkov eventually reveals that Russia has a state-sponsored Olympic doping program that he oversees."

that he ran a state-sponsored doping program for the Russians. The result was a full-fledged, totally-filmed whistle-blow on the Soviet's Olympic doping program. No one (particularly the film-maker) saw that coming.

In some sense, this sort of plot twist happened with *Invisible Scars*. Bob and his team *thought* they were "just" creating a documentary about PTSD. Along the way, though, they continued bumping into something known as Moral Injury.

"It looks like PTSD at first glance," many professionals and service providers said, "but the same treatment protocols don't help. It's clearly *not* PTSD." And, "If you treat it like PTSD, it doesn't work. You've got to do something else."

Others observed, "Sometimes, you find them together- both PTSD and Moral Injury. But they're different."

MI looks like PTSD at first glimpse because the symptoms- the externals (the "fruit")- manifests in common expressions. Notice the following graphic:

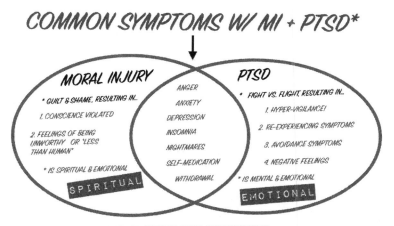

COMMON SYMPTOMS W/ MI + PTSD*

MORAL INJURY

* GUILT & SHAME, RESULTING IN...

1. CONSCIENCE VIOLATED

2. FEELINGS OF BEING UNWORTHY OR "LESS THAN HUMAN"

* IS SPIRITUAL & EMOTIONAL

SPIRITUAL

ANGER
ANXIETY
DEPRESSION
INSOMNIA
NIGHTMARES
SELF-MEDICATION
WITHDRAWAL

PTSD

* FIGHT VS. FLIGHT, RESULTING IN...

1. HYPER-VIGILANCE!

2. RE-EXPERIENCING SYMPTOMS

3. AVOIDANCE SYMPTOMS

4. NEGATIVE FEELINGS

* IS MENTAL & EMOTIONAL

EMOTIONAL

* BOTH ARE EXPRESSED IN SIMILAR EMOTIONAL WAYS!

In-depth interviews with soldiers, their family members, and additional professionals revealed that what they kept hearing to be true was, indeed, true. **Different than PTSD, Moral Injury is a real issue. Not only that, it's *deep*.**

In time (and through many conversations) it became apparent a follow-up film was needed. So, in 2016 Crosswinds released *Honoring the Code*, a film addressing issues of Moral Injury (which you may not yet have heard of) and Survivor's Guilt (which you probably have heard about).[53]

The short version is this: ***Moral Injury most often occurs when your conscience is violated.***

Think back to Dr. Perkus' "Three Facts About Human Nature" we discussed in Chapter 4:

- Fact #1 = we're designed to explore and grow.

- Fact #2 = as we explore we bump into things which cause us pain, something we want to avoid.

- Fact #3 = we create internal rules- often subconsciously to help us manage the tension between Facts #1 and #2.

Turns out, **there's also "human code" that's hardwired into the far, vast majority of us- a set of subconscious rules.** C.S. Lewis, the English professor who wrote *The Chronicles of Narnia*, likened it to a moral compass. Theologians refer to is as the image of God and the "law" that's written on our hearts. Whatever you call it, there are certain rules that are common across all cultures, all people groups, and virtually all times in history.

---

[53] Stream this second film at www.WarriorHope.com/HTC.

Everyone knows, even subconsciously, without being taught-

- Murder is wrong

- Lying, cheating, and stealing aren't right

- Rape and sexual assault are unacceptable

- Men should defer to and honor women, children, and the elderly

In other words, **we come hardwired with a set of rules**. When we break these rules, even if we've never been told not to, we feel deep internal unrest. We feel pain. We may even feel *broken*.

Why?

Because each of us have a conscience which actively communicates with us. Moreover, that conscience connects to the deepest, richest part of us, our spirit.

YOUR MORAL COMPASS

Webster's Dictionary defines *conscience* as,

> *the sense or consciousness of the moral goodness or blameworthiness of one's own conduct, intentions, or character together with a feeling of obligation to do right or be good.*

In general, here's how the conscience tends to affect people:

- If you know to do right but do the opposite the result may be a guilty conscience.

- If you know right but observe someone else do the opposite without trying to stop it, the result may be a guilty conscience.

- If you do what is right, the result should be a clear conscience.

In other words, if you put a gag on the voice of "do right" you will most likely experience a sense of guilt- even if you have no choice but to remain silent. **Sometimes this is a misplaced guilt as the "wrong" committed is not your fault- it could be something someone else did or it could be something was done to you- or wasn't actually a wrong.**

Some people think of the conscience as that inner voice which helps us distinguish right from wrong, like a "moral compass." Others believe it springs forth from our inner being (from our spirit or soul), giving it more of a "religious" or "spiritual" connection.

You may have seen the conscience depicted as an angel and a devil with one sitting on each shoulder of a person, whispering in their ear. The angel tells us to do right; the devil tells us to do wrong.

MORAL INJURY DEALS WITH OUR CONSCIENCE*

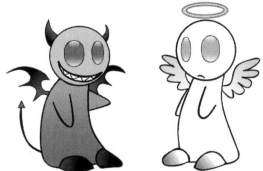

*IT OCCURS WHEN WE GO AGAINST OUR INTERNAL CODE OF ETHICS

One of the professionals featured in *Honoring the Code*, Dr. Rita Brock, offers incredible insight here. To better understand this issue, consider the causes and consequences of Moral Injury (MI) she identifies.

1.   Violating or going against one's core moral beliefs, one's conscience (this may be a personal choice or, as is the case soldiers often experience, one demanded or ordered by someone in authority).

2.   Evaluating one's behavior (actions) negatively *to the extent they can no longer think of themselves as a decent human being.*

Notice her second point. PTSD most often occurs when a person experiences, witnesses, or encounters a traumatic event. Though PTSD (even if undiagnosed) makes us feel uneasy, the issue often remains "out there." We can separate ourselves from it. MI, on the other hand, becomes so intertwined in the soul that we begin questioning our decency as humans.

The expression of the two is often different. **Whereas PTSD creates a "flight or fight" response (attack the issue that's "out there" or run away from it), MI typically manifests as overwhelming feelings of guilt or shame.**

You've probably heard the saying, "Wherever you go, there you are." When the issue is "in you" (i.e., your conscience), you can't fight it or run from it. It remains present at all times.

Earlier in the book we talked about perceptions and reality- and how PTSD (or any emotional trauma) affects both our mindset and our emotions. We think one thing is happening in the present (based on our past experience), so we sometimes react inappropriately.

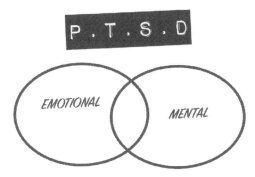

Is often characterized by a FIGHT vs. FLIGHT response.

Moral Injury is different. Whereas PTSD primarily deals with our mind and our emotions, MI primarily deals with our mind and our spirit.

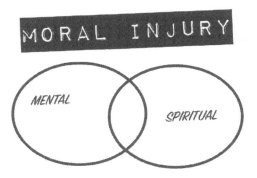

Is often characterized by feelings of GUILT and SHAME.

To be clear, our emotions can be involved with MI and our spirits can be involved with PTSD. These are each parts of our soul. Anything having to do with any part of us can affect every part of us. But, these simplistic graphics help provide a general framework to distinguish the two.

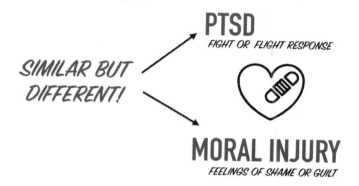

Furthermore, since PTSD and MI are two different issues, they must must be addressed in a much different matter. **PTSD must be addressed as being primarily a mental and emotional issue while MI, though it may have an emotional component, is basically a moral or spiritual issue.**

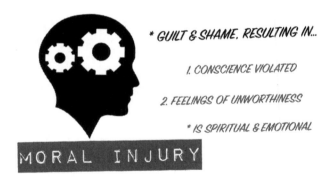

Earlier in the book I told you about a first responder-friend who, by his own admission, carried a weight of survivor's guilt. Remember, the man who trained him died one day while taking a routine call while my friend was scheduled "off" from work.

"It messed me up," he said. And- "I should have been there to stop it. Or it should have been me."

As he spoke more about his feelings related to the loss of a close co-worker, he described tangible guilt and unworthiness. In my opinion, he wasn't dealing with PTSD, he was sorting through Moral Injury. Remember, whereas PTSD elicits the "fight or flight" response, Moral Injury is accompanied by a sense of guilt and/or shame.

For a moment, let's separate the two concepts of guilt (what we do) and shame (who we are). The two, though related, are different. And this helps explain why MI is so devastating.

Whereas **guilt focuses on actions (what we do), shame declares identity (who we are).** People can repent of actions, but they can't repent of their identity.

Like we discussed earlier (chapters 5 & 6), an identity change requires we do more than rewrite the script. To change an identity we must re-cast the character. Or, to say it another way, we must address the *root causes* rather than looking at the *fruit symptoms.*

GUILT & SHAME COMPARISON

	BASED ON	DESCRIBED IN DETAIL
Guilt	Action- "I did something"	Something you do- it may be out of character for you, or could have been based on circumstances
Shame	Identity- "I am something"	Who you are- it's different than doing a "bad thing." This denotes you're a bad person, perhaps not even valued as a human

UNDIAGNOSABLE SKELETONS

Here's the strange thing about MI: everywhere I talk about it, as many people resonate with it as they do PTSD. By that, I mean this:

- In the same way most of us are not diagnosable with PTSD, understanding it helps us navigate our own emotional wounds. Most of us do not have Moral Injury, but we do struggle with feelings of guilt and shame.

- We see something tangible that we connect with- even though what we see, sense, or feel in our own lives may not be as extreme as the full-blown psychological condition. Seeing the "outlier" provides language for us whereby we can understand our own experience.

- Based on what we learn, we find ourselves more equipped to step towards overall health. The goal remains not to receive or reject a diagnosis, either way; the goal remains living whole.

Here's the kicker, though: **no one can currently be diagnosed with MI. It's not included in the DSM-5, which provides the basis for receiving any diagnosis.**[54]

But then again, remember, our goal isn't to get diagnosed (nor is it to avoid a diagnosis). Our goal is to walk in total health. That is, we want to define where we are, so we can walk into who we're designed to be.

---

[54] The current DSM-5 was a 2013 update. Many professionals believe Moral Injury will be in the DSM-6.

NOT AS BAD AS BOOKER

You probably don't have a story like Booker's. Few people do. Your story may be something more like this…

A few years ago I met a friend for coffee every Tuesday evening at 8:30pm (right after we tucked our kids in bed and had time to make a quick drive to the nearby Starbucks). It was our weekly 1:1 "small group."

One evening, he told me needed to get something off his chest. It was something he'd done a long time ago, something he'd never told anyone- not even his wife.

"What's up?" I asked.

"A few years ago, I _____."

He *completely* filled in the blank, telling me in a few short paragraphs the situation, the sin, and the strangle-hold which the secret held on him since the event he was hiding first happened.

I thought for a moment. Then I looked at him.

"*Is that it?* Is this what you've been carrying?" I expected something more, a somewhat bigger reveal. I mean, what he told me wasn't a "small" issue. It was significant, but the shame he expressed disproportionally outweighed the guilt of what he had done.

Immediately, I learned two things.

The first is that **the power of hidden secrets grows exponentially the longer we keep them dead-bolted behind closed doors**. No matter how big they are, and no matter how much we fear sharing them, the sooner we release them the easier.

The second is that, like we discussed with emotional wounds, **the size and scope of sin is often in the eyes of the beholder.** Don't misunderstand me. Wrong is wrong. But for various reasons, it affects each of us differently.

In the end, comparing one person's moral high ground to another person's low is a lot like comparing the summit of Everest to the depth of the abyss in the Pacific... from the Moon. The other day I heard that the surface of the earth is proportionally to its size smoother than an eight ball. Though the differences look radically disparate from here, grace heals them all the same.

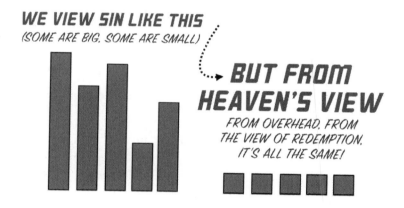

WE VIEW SIN LIKE THIS
(SOME ARE BIG, SOME ARE SMALL)

⟶ BUT FROM HEAVEN'S VIEW
FROM OVERHEAD, FROM THE VIEW OF REDEMPTION, IT'S ALL THE SAME!

I told him, "I'm sorry you've been weighted by this. That was then. You're free from it. I know who you really are. God forgives you. Set it down and don't pick it back up."

"I think I can now," he said. Then- "It seemed bigger when it was inside me."

Don't get me wrong. It wasn't a trite little thing he revealed. It's just that, well, in his words, "I guess I needed to let that skeleton out of the closet. He seemed scary when he was in there. Turns out, this whole time, he was just bones leaning up against that closed door, threatening to come out and pounce me."

I listened a moment, soaking his words. At that point, I had secrets, too.

He continued, "I just opened the door to you, afraid of what that skeleton would do to me when I did. But he didn't do anything. He just collapsed on the floor. He didn't have any strength at all."

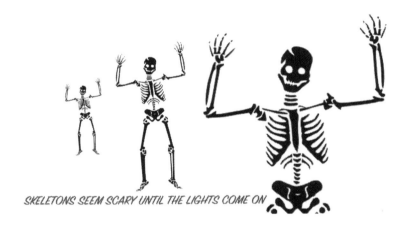

SKELETONS SEEM SCARY UNTIL THE LIGHTS COME ON

"No," I replied, as if to coach myself about releasing my own skeletons, about yanking them out of the closets where I'd shoved them away, out of sight but not out of mind. Then- "Skeletons don't have any muscle. No voice, either- so they can't accuse."

"They can't stand up or do anything on their own..."

"We're afraid of the light until we actually get there," I added. "Then we find it's the safest, easiest, most life-giving place to be."

It's scary, but it's *safe*.

The problem, of course, is that it can seem like a *long* way to get there. Whereas flipping a light switch in your house instantly pushes all the dark away, virtually eliminating the shadows in a moment (and confirming that no monsters live in the closet, under the bed, or any other tucked-away place), flipping the light on in life seems more like a process.

In a word, here's why: *fear*.

Again, even if the light is the safest place to be, it's also the most vulnerable and frightening. **Our timidity about being exposed has to do not only with what we've experienced but *who we think we are and who others will think we are*** because of what we've done, what was done to us, or what we failed to do.

Turn the page. There's a simple cure, but it's used far too little in comparison to the powerful potential it has to revolutionize, well… *everything*.

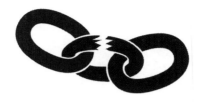

10. The All-Too-Uncommon Cure

For years I was afraid to talk about some of my struggles- some of the things that had happened to me as well as some of the things I had done. I was certain that I would be written off, rejected, abandoned.

It's a longer story than I'll write here, but as a result of my experience I decided I would provide safe space where no one in my closest sphere of influence would feel (as much as was possible on my end) afraid to approach me with the skeletons they had in their closet like I had been afraid to approach others before. I wanted to embody grace.

Contemplating *how* to do that led me to 1 John 4:18, a verse I pondered over and over for almost a solid year. It's a passage I'm trying to implement in my interpersonal relationships, in my writing, and from any stage or platform from which I speak. Further, it has everything to do with the "cure" for that guilt-shame duo we discussed in the previous chapter.

Here are two translations of the verse-

> There is no fear in love, but **perfect love casts out fear**. For fear has to do with punishment, and whoever fears has not been perfected in love (ESV).

And,

> Love never brings fear, for fear is always related to punishment. But **love's perfection drives the fear of punishment far from our hearts.** Whoever walks constantly afraid of punishment has not reached love's perfection (Passion).

Over the next few pages I want to highlight three concepts from the verse:

1.   Perfect love

2.   Casts out fear

3.   Fear reveals that we've not yet been perfected in love

Then we'll wrap it with a bow and resolve the Moral Injury issue- on paper, at least.

LOVE TO YOUR MAX POTENTIAL

First, let's define what "perfect" means. The word used in this passage doesn't infer we'll always love each other "without flaw." Rather it suggests we will love each other *maturely*, to the full capacity that we can love.

The Greek word "perfect" is *telios*. It doesn't mean "without error" (as we most often use the word *perfect*). Rather, it means "reaching full potential."

We find the word in Colossians 1:28, where Paul says,

> Him we preach, warning every man and teaching every man in all wisdom, that we may present every man **perfect** [telios] in Christ Jesus.

John, who also wrote in Greek like Paul, places the same word here in 1 John 4:18.[55] So, **he writes about a love that "reaches the full potential." Or, "fulfills the purpose for which it was created."**

In the same way Paul longed for his congregants to live their purpose and reveal their potential on a personal level, John wants us to "love our purpose." That is, **he wants our love to be whole, complete, and full of life.** Since the Spirit indwells us in His fullness, that is our capacity- to deliver the very heart of the Father to the world in which we live.

What does that kind of love look like?

Well, read the verse again. John describes it. A *telios* love pushes fear out and makes massive space for grace.

A la 1 Corinthians 13, *telios* love hopes for the best, believes the best, and never fails- even when the person being loved clearly falters (13:4f.). In fact, this love keeps *no record* of wrongs at all. It actually endures and abounds all the more aggressively when sin is present (see Romans 6:1). ***Telios* love is the antidote for hard things.**

EXPELS FEAR LIKE A DEMON

Second, let's discuss what "casts out fear" means. John tells us that mature love- the love that reaches its full potential- dominates fear. It doesn't incite fear or insecurity; it eliminates it. As such, ***telios* love makes people feel safe.**

---

[55] The New Testament was written in Greek and Aramaic.

I reviewed several translations to see how they translate the term "casts out." Here are four ways translators describe what perfect, *telios*, love does.[56]

- Drives out fear (NIV)

- Expels all fear (NLT)

- Casts out fear (ESV)

- Banishes fear (ISV)

In other words, this kind of love is *strong*- one of the most powerful forces in the universe. It's more potent than PTSD. It's more massive that Moral Injury. It shudders shame.

Here's how intensely it creates security: **the same word used of "casts out" fear is the same verbiage used throughout the New Testament to describe how Jesus treated demons.** When He bumped into them, they had no choice but to leave. He expelled them. He forced them to go. He eliminated them.

It's a great analogy. **Mature love- the God kind of love- does the exact same thing to condemnation, fear, and shame**. Perfect love drives fear away with this same passion. Fear has *no choice* but leave when people are loved in this way.

Now pause. Step back. Do a heart check. Let's be honest.

This *is the exact opposite* of what many people experience when they come in contact with our moral systems of right and wrong, our religious routines, and our beliefs systems about "making the world a better place." Rather than driving fear

---

56 NIV = New International Version, NLT = New Living Translation, ESV = English Standard Version, ISV = International Standard Version

away from the relationship and communicating, "Hey, come in close... tell me what's really happening..." we often *invite fear* and place it on the person like a cloak of shame. **They already feel devastated, yet we often want to make them feel *more* morally broken as we think that will safeguard them from breaking that universal subset of Fact #3 rules again.**

Seems odd once you put it on paper and take a logical look at it, doesn't it?!

I've done it in parenting, I've done it in preaching, I've done it in relationships. We often *like* it when others have a "healthy" measure of fear, because it allows us to control the interaction and maintain the upper hand. We're afraid that if they don't experience some degree of fear, they might not see how desperately they need grace. They might not change. They might not "get their stuff together." We might not be able to control them.

But think practically about the environment surrounding Jesus...

- Tax collectors not only felt comfortable talking with Him, they felt confident enough in His love to invite their wayward friends to a party at which He would be present (Matthew 9:9-13).[57]

- Women who earned their money in licentious ways knew He would receive them. They were so certain they would be accepted by Him that they barged into dinners where they weren't invited (see Luke 7:36f.).[58]

---

[57] This episode is interesting, as it's the first time in which we see Jesus dining with "tax collectors and sinners." When asked why He does this, He explains that people who are well don't need a physician- just people who are sick (9:12). And, He calls the Pharisees to exercise mercy, as opposed to sacrifice (see Hosea 6:6, also).

[58] Judas objected to the lavish waste of money on the oils. Think about where the money came from? How does a woman of the street earn enough money to possess a container of oil worth "a year's wages" for a common laborer?

- Lepers- people the Law demanded stay away from others- actually approached Jesus so that He might touch them (Mark 1:40f.).[59]

- Roman soldiers, those who occupied the Jewish areas like warlords, keeping Jesus and His people in physical subservience, were able to look beyond the *Us vs. You* dilemma and approach Him for personal needs (Matthew 8:5f.). Jesus commended and rewarded their great faith.

- People considered "unclean" and excluded from the Temple (like the women with the flow of blood)- and believed to be *so unclean* that they would make others ceremonially unclean by touching them- boldly moved through crowds and *touched* Jesus (Mark 5:25f.).[60] They *knew* they would be embraced.

- Religious leaders approached Him, too- men like Jairus, whose daughter was at death's door (Mark 5:22f.). He abandoned protocol and knelt before Jesus publicly, imploring Him to visit her. And Nicodemus, one of the elite Pharisees who came to Him at night and asked how a person could be "born again" (John 3:1f.).

Notably, *most* of these people carried some obvious skeleton that stood in direct opposition to a specific Scriptural command. Most of them had been shunned because of it. Yet, despite that, they all felt safe with Jesus.

---

[59] A leper should not have greeted Jesus with, "If You are willing you can make me clean." According to religious tradition and custom, the leper should have cautioned Jesus to stay away from him, because of his ailment.

[60] According to Leviticus 15:25f., this woman *could* have made Jesus "unclean" by touching Him. He would have been unclean until the evening, potentially.

Are these the people who feel welcome near us? Or would they be afraid to approach us, because we haven't been perfected in love?

FEAR OF BEING CALLED-OUT, PUNISHED, HUMILIATED

Third, finally, let's discuss why people are afraid, that is, why they keep the wounds of the past bottled up. John, who spent three years with Jesus and was present at each of the encounters mentioned above, provides us with a clue. After telling us *"telios* love expels fear" he clearly explains *why* people fear.

He writes, "Fear involves punishment" (1 John 4:18).

In each of the instances above, **people who approached Jesus *knew* they'd find themselves pulled closer rather than pushed away and punished**, *regardless of how big and horrific the issue was, right?*

They didn't need to self-protect. They didn't need to preserve their dignity. They didn't need to hide behind a veil. He elevated them higher than they'd *ever* been, even as many of them brought their biggest shame and disappointment to Him.

In another verse in the same chapter, John writes (1 John 4:12 NLT),

> *No one has ever seen God. But if we love each other, God lives in us and His love is brought to full expression in us.*

Notice what John says. Even though none of us have physically seen our Redeemer, **we tangibly experience the complete manifestation of who**

He is when we encounter unconditional love from another human. *That* is when we feel safe to be completely exposed and vulnerable.

Only *that kind* of love works. In fact, that is the kind of love that shreds fear and shame, truly breathing life into people.

Imperfect, immature love does the exact opposite. It instills fear, it creates hiding, it empowers shame. It focuses on the rules rather than the relationship; it values written letters over love in action.

I can't imagine the atrocities of war. I've never been.

An elderly gentleman who served as the librarian at a church I attended during seminary was flabbergasted when *Saving Private Ryan* hit the big screen back in 1998. Whereas critics and "commoners" like me praised its graphic depiction of the battlefront, he had a different take all together.

"It's not real," he said. "Everything I saw in Normandy was 7 or 8 times worse. The air was dirty. There were people falling next to you in gory ways the films can *never* depict. The colors were different. The sound was deafening, and the smell was something I'd never experienced…"

I stood there, his words engulfing me.

He continued. "I hope people never see what it's *really* like. It's horrific. War is hell on earth."

My naive, 24-year-old self wondered what could possibly be more graphic than *Saving Private Ryan*. I couldn't envision it, no matter how hard I tried. I just listened.

After a few moments, he added- **"I don't know that people around here would look at me the same way if they know what that was really like, the things I experienced, and the things I had to do."**

There it was. *Bullseye.*

Not just emotional wounds, but spiritual wounds. Moral damage. Moral Injury.

Something had stung his soul in the deepest way. He wasn't "fighting" or "flighting," as is the case with PTSD. He carried guilt and shame. And this brave soldier who stared Hitler eye-to-eye was afraid of church people.

"Would we look *at you* the same?" I asked.

"Yes. All of that destruction you see on the film, and everything that happened during the War... *that was done by people.* By soldiers. By young men like me."

Sadly, I never thought about that conversation again after that until I began writing this chapter. In my mind, we *had* accepted him. He was the church librarian. He was "one of us."

But in his mind, he wasn't. He always carried around the baggage of things he held back- a skeleton in the closet that seemed infinitely scarier the longer it remained propped behind closed doors.

He was afraid that if he revealed that skeleton, we would shun him. Growing up in a religious environment, he'd probably seen enough evidence to verify that, yes, shunning happens. Sure, **we cloak it in "acceptable" language, but we still do it. We shame people into silence about their biggest secrets, their deepest hurts.**

As I began writing *Warrior Hope*, working my way back through the *Invisible Scars* and *Honoring the Code* documentaries, and sitting across the table from numerous veterans of all ages, I heard the same refrain from many of them.[61]

"I'm not so sure what my family would think of me if they knew the things I did over there."

And- "If people understood how many things I had to do that I never thought I would ever do…"

Or, "I feel like there's a *me* from over there that I would like to leave there, and I feel like there's a *me* now. There's a tension between those two…"

In other words, they're afraid they won't be accepted.

WHAT IT HAS TO DO WITH MORAL INJURY

All that said, let's talk about what this has to do with Moral Injury (MI).

MI occurs when the experiences or choices a person makes (or is exposed to, even through no fault of their own), conflicts with their personal code of conduct, morals, or ethics– the things we hold as right and wrong. As you can imagine, anyone struggling with this will feel great guilt and/or shame. I just relayed what I've heard from soldiers, but the mantra is the same from people who experience MI *for any reason*.

---

61 Stream these free at InvisibleScars.online and WarriorHope.com/HTC.

Let me tell you what the data reveals- and, I promise, you'll understand why the 80% of this chapter seemed more like a Bible study than a chapter in a book about freedom. It seems like a simple answer, but the data is *consistent*. **Practitioners of healing who study MI– from both secular sources and sacred sources – agree that overcoming MI requires one thing...**

You can't bottle it. You can't package it. You can't mass-deliver it.

The all-too-uncommon cure for Moral Injury is *receiving forgiveness* from someone the wounded person believes has the moral authority to grant that forgiveness.

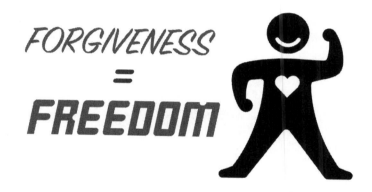

They need to hear the words "You're forgiven. You're accepted. It's the past."

Some even need to hear "I'm proud of the person you are."

And others even need the words "I love you."

Who has such authority to gift these words?

It depends on the person who needs it. It might be:

- A pastor, a priest, or a rabbi

- A former coach

- An officer or soldier someone served with- or even people who served that they don't know personally

- Someone else they perceive as an authority

It *must* be someone they believe, sense, or feel has the authority to impart forgiveness. It is at this point the healing process often begins.

I know. **You might have been looking for a more revelatory answer- for seven steps, a weekend retreat, a pilgrimage, or something akin to** *doing something* **significant rather than** *receiving something* **significant.**

If you come from a faith tradition like me, you might have just winced a bit when I suggested that coaches and soldiers and teachers and anyone else can dispense forgiveness. I know, that sounds strange.

But then there's this…

During Jesus' ministry, the Pharisees regularly scolded Him for forgiving people.[62] In their mind, only God could do that.

In response, at the end of His time on earth, Jesus did something incredibly interesting. We find it in John 20.

After they discovered the empty tomb, the disciples hid in the Upper Room- afraid they might be killed, too. **Jesus appeared to them behind the locked doors,**

---

[62] See Mark 2:7, for instance.

showing that our emotional duress (i.e., even fear itself) doesn't hinder Him from finding us.

John tells us He breathed the Holy Spirit upon them.

Then, He declared, "If you forgive the sins of any, they are forgiven them; if you withhold forgiveness from any, it is withheld" (John 20:23 ESV).

Clearly, **He expanded the power of imparting forgiveness farther and wider than the religious elite of the day dreamed possible.** Not only could God in Heaven forgive sins, but His Son certainly could (Mark 2:10-11). And not only could *that* Son forgive sins, but *all* the King's sons and daughters could.

Perhaps this is why Jesus said that "all men will know you are My disciples… by the way you love one another" (see John 13:34-35).

Love communicates something nothing else can. **Love is the greatest revelation possible to an unbelieving or desperately-wanting-to-believe world**. Love creates sacred space where much-needed healing happens.

(And, remember, sacred and secular professionals alike agree that freedom is found in forgiveness.)

IF THAT DESCRIBED YOU

If you're suffering with guilt or shame, let me remind you that you can always find a story to back your perception that you'll be rejected. I revealed the most to the person I loved the best and was shunned the hardest. And, like the vet in the church library, I've learned that some of the biggest offenders of loving people imperfectly are the most oblivious to it, even using pop psychology, Bible verses, and well-worn phrases that sound more cliché than real.

But that's not the norm. Most people want to dispense grace because, at the core, they know that they've needed it before and will need it again.

Freedom is always found on the other side of transparency. Perhaps you need to let go of things you've done. Or you need to release the weight of things you've experienced- things that were done to you or things that you witnessed firsthand. Whatever the case, freedom is found in the light.

Label it. Light it up. Let it go…

Yet, remember that not everyone needs access to your story. You may decide to talk to more people in the future, but freedom in the area you're hiding begins the instant you talk to "the few" we talked about in the intro.

Turn the page. In the next chapter we'll discuss what to do next, to continue moving forward. **Freedom isn't just about dealing with the past, it's about letting go of who you were so that you can live as the person you're designed to be.** That is, freedom has a future orientation as well.

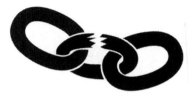

11. Therapeuo for Emotional Health = More Freedom Tools

By now, you know my bias: I prop on Scripture and do my best to lean into the Spirit. No problem here if you don't- we can disagree, still interact with each other, and learn a lot together.

Since this is my book, though, and we've already "gone there," let me show you something else from the Bible. This will apply to you, too, even if that's not your chosen belief system. Since you've been with me for 170 pages, give me a bit of grace and work through the next few. It will be worth it, I promise.

That said, there are multiple words we find in the New Testament for *healing*. In this chapter I want to teach you two of them, as they have everything to do not only with physical health + healing but also emotional health + healing.[63]

---

[63] The New Testament was originally written in Greek and Aramaic. *Sozo* is a third word that sometimes references healing, as well.

Understanding *why* we find different are words in the Biblical text is important, as they each refer to different things. Let me explain…

One word for healing, *iaomai*, means "miraculous" or "instant change."
It's abrupt. It's cataclysmic. It changes things *immediately*.

We see *iaomai* throughout the New Testament:

- Jesus *iaomai* the blind man who had never, ever seen *anything* from the moment he was born (John 9:1f.)

- Jesus *iaomai* the paralytic who was lowered through the roof by four friends (Mark 2:1f.)

- Jesus *iaomai* the lame man at the Pool of Bethesda (John 5:1f.)

- Jesus *iaomai* the leper (Mark 1:40f.)

No one debates the fact that Jesus healed with miracles. Not even people from other faith traditions. In fact, when we think about *how* Jesus healed people, we all most often *exclusively* envision Him performing miracles.

Turns out, He still does miracles today. I've seen *iaomai* firsthand. In other books I've described my sister's heart murmur (completely healed), my brother's gouged eye (perfect vision) and my uncle's death at UAB (he's still alive, 20 years later). These are each examples of *iaomai*. Clearly, I believe Jesus healed in the past, and I believe He still heals in the present.

I tell you that because I want you to understand that I emphatically *don't* have an anti-miracle bias when I relay this next concept to you. (I've taught this info in a few charismatic churches who clearly think I do have anti-miracle bias.)

Here it is: *Whereas He performed miracles for some, Jesus also taught others to be well, to live a lifestyle of health and wholeness. That is, Jesus instructed people how to choose wellness.* [64]

The second word we see in the New Testament for "healing" is therapeuo. It means to "teach how to be well, to wait on, to heal over time." You might recognize its resemblance to our word *therapy*.

TWO WORDS FOR HEALING

WORD	APPEARS	MEANING	HAPPENS
iaomai	30 times	Instantaneous healing	Spontaneously, in the moment
therapeuo	40 times	To serve, to attend to, or to wait upon menially- even by teaching them to be well	Intentionally, over time

The word *iaomai* (instant healing) is used 30 times in the New Testament- and the word *therapeuo* (healing over time) is used 40 times. In other words, there may actually be a slight emphasis on the "walk it out over time" method of healing.

THEY WORK TOGETHER

We actually see *both* of these words working together in Matthew 8, a passage in which the former tax collector strings together a series of healing events as a

---

[64] We talk about this in more detail in the first book in our "Books You'll Actually Read Series," *Health + Healing & Essential Oils*. More info at www.OilyApp.com/books.

commentary on Isaiah 53- the passage that prophesied that the Messiah would be a healer.[65]

Matthew tells us Jesus healed several people instantly:

- A leper approached Him and was instantly made whole (8:3).

- A centurion's servant who'd contracted a disease that inflicted immediate paralysis on his body was healed (8:13).

- Peter's mother-in-law, who had been on her deathbed with an extreme fever, rose and began serving them as soon as Jesus touched her (8:15).

Clearly, Jesus *iaomai* people.

Matthew tells us that this series of three miracles created such a pleasant commotion that the entire village gathered together at Peter's mother-in-law's house after learning she was well. Anyone who was sick or demon possessed was immediately brought to Him for attention.

Matthew then tells us, "He healed them with a word" (8:16).

I used to read that passage and emphasize the "with a word" part- as if Jesus simply spoke and something supernaturally magical happened.

"Here, you be healed!"

Then, "You, too. Go your way and be merry."

And, "Also, you... right there. In the back. You, as well."

---

65 "He was pierced for our transgressions. He was crushed for our iniquities. Upon Him was the chastisement that brought us peace, and with His stripes we are healed" (Isaiah 53:5 ESV).

Obviously, Jesus did that kind of thing. Matthew just showed us a series of three encounters where that type of thing happened.

Yet here, in this verse (8:16), Matthew reports that something else occurred altogether. Yes, Jesus healed them, but the word Matthew uses to denote that He did isn't the word *iaomai*. Rather, it's the word *therapeuo*.

Matthew *literally* tells us that, when the crowds rallied together at Peter's MIL's house, Jesus "healed" them by "teaching them how to live well." Furthermore, Matthew includes *this* in his treatise on the Isaiah 53 passage!

He concludes this series of healing events by penning (Matthew 8:17):

> *This was to fulfill what was spoken through the prophet Isaiah: "He took up our infirmities and bore our diseases."*

In other words, **healing people *instantly* and healing people *over time* by teaching them to live well are *both* aspects of what Jesus came to do.**

Sometimes, Jesus heals instantly. Other times, He teaches people how to be well. Sometimes, Jesus touches us and we are dramatically changed in that moment. Other times, He imparts His wisdom to us so that we can "walk out" the freedom.[66]

Now, think about what this *really* means, practically. Let's move it from theory to real life:

- Jesus can heal lung cancer, but He can also teach us about the ills of smoking.

- He can cure diabetes. He also shows us how to eat better.

---

[66] Find examples in Matthew 4:23-24, Mark 1:34, Mark 6:13, Luke 5:15, Acts 5:16, Acts 8:7, Revelation 22:2.

- He can heal sexually transmitted diseases. He also provides us with directions on how to live whole and healthy lives, as well as experience the joy of true intimacy with one person.

- He can heal us of the dozens of physical nuisances that we've grown to tolerate. Or, we can take His directions and experience what it really means to be alive!

Let me show you another example and then we'll apply it to emotional and mental health.[67]

AND YET AGAIN

The story begins in Acts 27. Paul, Luke, and 274 other travelers find themselves shipwrecked on the island of Malta.[68]

Luke, the traveler reporting the story, was a well-known physician. Furthermore, he's the New Testament author that communicates the most thoroughly about the Holy Spirit and God's supernatural power to perform miracles. This is an important detail, because it shows us he'll be balanced and honest with the data-

- As a physician, he'll tell us if healthy lifestyle choices were involved

- As a miracle-worker, he'll tell us if God intervened and did something we can't humanly explain

---

[67] Matthew's explanation that Jesus "taught people to be well" isn't an isolated instance in the Bible. In fact, we see this trend throughout the New Testament.

[68] See Acts 27:36.

Both sides of the equation are important. Remember, Jesus *did* both.

The shipwrecked crew made their way to the shore and built a fire to warm themselves. In the hustle, they stirred a snake pit. After surviving a viper bite that should have killed him instantly, the islanders concluded Paul had a supernatural reason for being there. In fact, they perceived him to be a god (see Acts 28:6, and remember that entire perception-reality tango we discussed in chapter 2).

Luke writes that, because of this, Paul was taken to the local chief, who was confined to this deathbed, most likely with a dreaded illness like dysentery (Acts 28:7-9). Luke details that Paul *iaomai* him. To use language we're familiar with, *this was a miracle.*

The remainder of the islanders gathered to the hut after this encounter, much in the same way that the crowds flocked to Jesus after He healed Peter's MIL. Luke, who would know *exactly* what happened from the vantage point of being both an eyewitness and a skilled medical professional (as well as a man who understood the powerful potential of the Holy Spirit), explains that Paul then healed *every* diseased person on the island (Acts 28:9). To be clear, Paul *therapeuo* the entire island. That is, *he taught them how to live well.*

Or, to say it another way, those were *not* miracles.

WHAT GOD DOES, WHAT YOU DO

When I teach the concepts above, I most often define my terms at the beginning of the class, talk, or lecture. It keeps everyone on the same page and eliminates the guesswork.

I usually say something like, "When I say the word *healing*, I'm referring to miracles, to *iaomai*, to something God does. We might pray and ask Him to do it, but it's something that- unless He does it- doesn't happen."

I often add, "In fact, He *has* to do it. I can't. So, I'm not going to take the credit if He does it, and I won't take the blame if He doesn't. I'll ask Him, but that's where it sits…"

Most people instantly understand that definition. And they realize that, "Yes, this is something God does."

So, I move to the next concept: "When I say the word *health*, I'm referring to choices you make that support wholeness and wellbeing. This is *therapeuo*. This is something you do."

Most people understand that, too.

What many people have *not* understood before is that they don't have to choose between one or the other. In fact, both are important. Each on enhances the other. Jesus did both. Paul did both. We can, too.[69]

HEALTH & HEALING

WORD	WHAT	WHO DOES IT	IS A...
Healing	*iaomai*	Something God does	Miracle
Health	*therapeuo*	Something you do	Lifestyle

---

[69] I outline each of these words- and the definitions I use- at the beginning of *Health + Healing & Essential Oils*, book 1 in our series. More info at www.OilyApp.com/books.

CONTROL WHAT YOU CAN CONTROL

A few years ago I read that cancer is 90-95% connected to environmental factors and only 5-10% related to genetics. I read it on a government website- not an obscure site about "all things natural health only." Look-

> Only 5–10% of all cancer cases can be attributed to genetic defects, whereas the remaining 90–95% have their roots in the environment and lifestyle.[70]

In other words, we may have far more control over that dreaded disease than we once thought. We're not victims of genetics, helpless and hopeless apart from a miracle. Turns out, we have far more control over most health issues than we've previously thought.

When I teach these concepts, I usually tell people, "Yes, let's pray for a miracle. Let's hope that happens. I have faith that it can."

We pray, and often miracles come.

I always tell them, too, "Even if a miracle doesn't happen, we're going to start walking in health right now, though."

That is, we're going to immediately make lifestyle adjustments that stand in line with overall health and wholeness. **Miracles, it seems, are needed for the 5% of things we can't control. Our choices can radically influence the other 95%.** If you begin making wise decisions, the odds are *radically* in your favor.

I conclude, "Miracle or no miracle, healing starts now."

---

[70] Source = https://www.ncbi.nlm.nih.gov/pmc/articles/PMC2515569/, accessed 07/02/2019.

By that, I mean this: If God does the thing that only He can do and we see a supernatural breakthrough, we receive it and celebrate. If, on the other hand, He doesn't, we still make healthy choices in alignment with what we want our bodies to do.

In fact, I encourage people to make those choices, *anyway*. I tell them that we want our lifestyle to always reflect our goals. If, for instance, cancer is 95% environmental and 5% genetic, we don't want to receive a miracle that heals the 5% and then not adjust the 95% of factors which we *can* control. We want all of our decisions to support what we've received.

Make sense?

WHAT THAT HAS TO DO WITH THIS

Jesus commanded His disciples- and empowered them- to preach the Gospel of the Kingdom when He sent them out. He told them to *heal* people as they did (Luke 9:2, for example).[71] Healing was clearly part of their message, part of the "total package" they carried wherever they went.

When Jesus sent out the 70, He said: "Heal the sick there, and say to them, 'The Kingdom of God has come near...'" (Luke 10:9).

I want you to notice the "kind" of healing He sent them to demonstrate and teach, though. This is *revelatory*.

The word He used, the word we translate as "heal," is *therapeuo*. Not *iaomai*.

---

71 They had to receive the healing, first- and then take it to others.

They weren't sent to *only* instantly heal people with miracles (which we know they did from other places throughout the New Testament). They were *also* told to teach a Kingdom way of life. That is, they were sent to show people how to live well, how to be whole.

Here's what all of that has to do with this book.

First, I want to empower you- as much as I possibly can- to live emotionally whole, to be well "from the inside-out." Earlier in the book we even discussed how sometimes getting the stuff "on the inside" right leaks to the outside and transforms it. It's highly likely that any issues you may have in your body will follow the condition of your soul.[72]

Second, emotional healing isn't just an instant-*iaomai*-miracle proposition; it's a lifestyle. Sure, I believe the Father *often* heals people in a moment- even of emotional wounds.

But, it's possible- and even highly probable- you'll find healing through the process of walking it out. Too many people wait to get struck by lightning, that is, for a supernatural event to occur that suddenly becomes their breakthrough.

What if that doesn't happen? Is all hope vanquished?

Of course not. We can still *therapeuo* our way there. We can claim our freedom and begin the process of sorting life and fighting for wholeness.

The Declaration of Independence was signed on July 4, 1776. We celebrate that day every year with fireworks, swimming, long days at the beach, and more. That is the day our Founding Fathers claimed our freedom.

---

72 See chapter 1, "Live Inside-Out Not Outside-In."

But we weren't yet free.

They claimed freedom before anyone saw the finality of it. You see, the military campaigns of the Revolutionary War lasted from 1775 until 1783. It took seven years of walking in a freedom that didn't yet exist in order to truly be free.

Don't miss the parallel. You might have to stake a claim and begin your freedom march before there's evidence, as well.

And, even if the miracle does happen, you're going to want to walk the lifestyle anyway, right?

TOOLS FOR MENTAL + EMOTIONAL WHOLENESS

For the final few pages of this chapter, I want to outline four things you can do right now- three of which are *free*- to walk in emotional health.

1. Eat better

2. Move more

3. Write it out

4. Seek professional help

As we placed a video on our website (login and watch it at www.OilyApp.com/Freedom) where we discuss these in more detail, I'll keep this brief.

First, eat better.

Scientists regularly refer to the gut "the second brain." Shaped much like your brain, your stomach features millions of neurons and possesses its own nervous system (which mirrors the system in your brain). Anything that happens "down there" impacts everything everywhere else in your body.

If you have kids, you've known this for years, haven't you?

Toss the little ones some broccoli and they remain calm. Sure, they may complain, but it's a docile whine at worst.

Toss them a bag of Sour Patch Kids (and a Capri Sun juice bag) and you'll see a different level of fury altogether. It's akin to unleashing the Kraken.[73]

Why?

Because anything that goes in the stomach radically affects the brain.

Let me offer you another tidbit about the gut: *Your stomach actually "thinks" on some level.* I know, that sounds weird, so hear me out.

You've probably had insight- or intuition- before and just known that something was really, really right or that something was a bit "off." If asked how you knew it, you might reply, "I just knew in my gut." In fact, you might not even be able to put it into words.

Another example…

You probably stepped into the unknown before- into a hard situation in which you had to be brave. You knew it was a stretch for you, marching through uncharted territory where you didn't know the outcome. But you pressed on. You may have

---

[73] https://en.wikipedia.org/wiki/Kraken

even felt "butterflies" in your stomach, alerting you to something that you- again- couldn't quite explain with words.

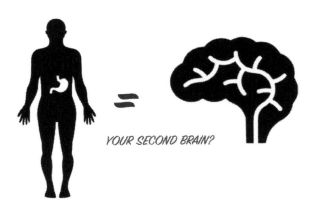

YOUR SECOND BRAIN?

When dealing with hard things, it makes sense to give your body the best fuel you can. In fact, it makes sense to do that *all of the time*, because when you get "gut health" right, many of the health issues we regularly juggle tend to actually sort themselves and resolve.

So...

- Eat more "live" foods (i.e., it grows in a garden or on a tree).

- Eat more protein (a lot of vegetables have protein, by the way, so you can achieve this even if you're a vegetarian).

- Stop eating processed foods, as well as anything that has any ingredient on the label that you can't pronounce.

Second, move more.

The next step you can take to walking in emotional *therapeuo* is to exercise. It sounds obvious, but many people- when feeling down- tend to slow way down physically and occupy themselves with other things (i.e., scrolling social media, binging Netflix, etc.). Enjoy a movie, sure, but don't stop moving.

Here are a three reasons why you need to move more-

Reason #1 = remember that tiredness mimics depression and depression mimics tiredness. Exercise, though, actually generates its own energy. So, when you move- even if it's just a 20-30 minute walk, you send your body sparking in the opposite direction.

Reason #2 = exercise is a neurological process that fires the left side of the brain. Whereas the right side of your brain is emotive and creative, the left side of the brain is the logical, rational hemisphere. Exercise, then, awakens the part of your mind that, by default, deals more with logic and reason rather than emotion.

For sure, both sides of the brain are important. But, when you're dealing with hard things it's important to not only feel them but to also work through them in an ordered way. "Waking" the left side of the brain helps you sort, file, and review as you move forward.

Reason #3 = exercise awakens your parasympathetic nervous system (as opposed to the sympathetic nervous system). Here's the difference:

> *Sympathetic is responsible for the response commonly referred to as "fight or flight," while parasympathetic is referred to as "rest and digest."*

> *... The sympathetic nervous system is the part of the autonomic nervous system*
> *that prepares the body to react to stresses such as threat or injury.*[74]

In other words, the sympathetic nervous system- by default- generates the survival instincts commonly exhibited in cases of PTSD.[75] The sympathetic nervous system can make you *feel* like you're dealing with stress- even if you're not.

The parasympathetic nervous system, on the other hand, is the opposite of stress. It puts your body at rest which- as you might remember- places us back in rhythm.[76]

Like I mentioned earlier, most of my best ideas emerge while I'm exercising- when my body and mind are free to just "be." My thoughts organize themselves, the chaos evaporates, and things begin making sense.

Plus, let's be honest, exercise makes you look better. And, often, just looking better automatically makes you feel better.

That said, let's discuss the next tool for walking in emotional wholeness.

Third, write it out.

This third one *always* trips people up.

"I'm not a writer," they say.

No worries. You don't have to be. You're not writing to publish, and you're not writing to leave a legacy journal behind for your kids. You're writing *for you*.

---

[74] Accessed from http://www.softschools.com/difference/sympathetic_vs_parasympathetic/143/ on 07/02/2019.

[75] See chapter 3, "The Goal = Health," for more about PTSD.

[76] Review chapter 8.

And by "writing" I mean actually *writing* with a pen (or pencil) and paper. *Not typing.*

Here's why: writing by hand is a neurological process that helps your mind do more of that sorting. Think about it for a moment. As I write this sentence, I'm mentally required to connect it to the previous sentence as well as the next one. My brain makes connections and builds relationships among various strands of thought on auto-pilot as I do.

(It sounds like this should work when you type, but it doesn't. It's completely different. As a writer, trust me. It is.)

Now, sorting a non-sense sentence like the one I just wrote isn't that important in the grand scheme of life. But, sorting past hurts, current problems, and future potential is incredibly important.

Plus, there are different kinds of writing-

- You can simply "mind-dump" and "bullet point" things onto paper, effectively off-loading them from your brain.

- You can journal your story like I did over the past year, effectively mapping your life in order to understand the patterns and gain perspective on the bigger picture.

- You can make a list of things you feel. Then, with some time and space, look at them objectively. Circle the ideas that are truths, thoughts you need to cling to. Scratch through ideas that are false beliefs, things where you've had the wrong perspective and need to let something go.

(JB is noted for doing the third, and then tossing the paper in the trash!)

In her book *Switch On Your Brain*, Dr. Caroline Leaf coaches her readers through a "21 Day Detox," in which they learn to recognize harmful thinking patterns from helpful ones, all while dealing with past hurts so that they might move forward full of hope.

Since it takes 60 days to create a new habit (even a mental habit, such as constructing a new thinking pattern), she suggests people complete the detox 3 times and then evaluate where they are. Her goal is to *automate* right thinking so that people can walk forward in emotional and mental health. In other words, **in the same way we can find ourselves *triggered* in destructive ways, we can also train ourselves to *trigger* our thoughts in helpful ways.**

How's that for neuro-hacking?

Every day we're bombarded with multiple mental and emotional grenades. Leaf reminds us, "You need to choose and decide whether or not these incoming thoughts will become part of who you are."[77]

She refers making right thinking the automatic "go to" as *automatization*.

She says, "If you don't practicing using it, it will not be properly automatized."[78]

And,

> … *Automatization means that particular way of thinking or reacting embedded in the new thought tree has become an automatic part of you; you do it driven by the non-conscious mind, not the conscious mind.*[79]

---

[77] *Switch on Your Brain*, p65.

[78] Caroline Leaf, *Switch On Your Brain*, p152.

[79] Caroline Leaf, *Switch On Your Brain*, p152.

The best way to automatize right thinking is... grasp this...by writing your thoughts on paper so that you can see them.

Fourth, seek professional help.

A few years ago I watched pastor Rick Warren, the iconic pastor responsible for penning *The Purpose Driven Life*, stand before an audience and talk openly about some of his family's struggles.

"A few years into our marriage, we went to marital counseling," he said. "We didn't see a way forward, so we sought outside help."

He said people always ask him how he afforded it. The *first* time (of many times) he sought counseling was well before his church was established, two decades before his books became best-sellers. He had a meager salary and no book deals or royalties.

"I put the counseling sessions on a credit card," he confessed. "I didn't have the money, and I knew we needed to go, so I just did what I would do if my car broke down and I had to get it fixed or if something at the house needed to be repaired and I couldn't afford it. I basically financed my therapy."

I'm not arguing you should go create a massive credit card bill- or even go into debt- to seek professional help. However, I do want to highlight two reasons you should consider professional help- from a financial perspective.

Reason #1 = we regularly seek professional help *for just about everything except emotional and mental wounds.* We hire professional trainers to rebuild our bodies, we hire CPAs to manage our money, and we pay architects to design our houses.

Why are we averse to hiring professionals to help us rebuild our souls, manage our thoughts & feelings, and renovate the life we want?

Reason #2 = we accept debt as a "given" for numerous other things.

Most people think *nothing* of financing a vehicle or a home. In fact, most people actually *choose* to do it that way. It's the accepted norm.

Why, then, are we averse to financing the cure of our souls?

Again, I'm not saying we should. I'm just, well… thinking out loud.

JB makes no bones about it. "After the dark stuff happened in my marriage, I went to counseling. Every day. For a long time. I wept, I learned things about me I needed to do, and we went deep. It was expensive, but it was worth it."

When he and Cindy lost Evans, he went to *more* counseling.

After he exploded his knee wave-boarding and found himself confined to a wheelchair for a year, growing more desperate and depressed by the day, he went to even *more* counseling.

Today, he walks in freedom and joy. In fact, he's so free that you're likely surprised when I tell you that he has "a past" that's chock full of pain.

How so?

He's confronted the skeletons- all of them. They've been revealed to have no muscle, no voice, no life left in them…

I'm still in process, but I'm learning **we'll only be as free as the past pain we're willing to confront.** Sometimes that requires help from an outside source, someone trained to do that heavy confrontation with us.

I know.

Firsthand.

Remember, I got that psych eval. And I had to be referred for it by a counselor.

After navigating the wiles of a traumatic adoption, learning of abuse in our home, and being gaslighted and shunned by a once-close confidant, I confronted the past head on.

I stormed the gates of hell with a water pistol.

Along the way, I experienced a few "miracles" and breakthroughs, sure. But, most of my freedom came as I *therapeuo'd* my way forward…

- I ate the right foods, avoiding binge eating and stress eating.

- I started moving again, running a bit less than I normally did and lifting less than I could, but creating space where I could be alone.

- I journaled 700-plus pages- with pen and ink. That activity alone, sometimes done for 3 or 4 hours a day, was difficult (I often teared-up, even while sitting in coffee shops and other public places) yet more freeing than any other activity I did. By putting things on paper I was able to not only see them, but my mind was able to make connections and help me see more clearly.

- I continued seeing a professional. His perspective helped me define terms and concepts and labels that are often misused in our culture, particularly by others who want to keep you down when you're at your lowest.

CHOOSING TO LIVE FREE

I learned… no, I'm *learning*… this, too: **Freedom is a choice. You must, as the title of this book says, *claim it*. Sometimes, you claim it before you can even see it as a possibility.**

And then you remind yourself of what you've chosen, even surrounding yourself with others who will serve as that voice for you. In fact, though I haven't addressed it in this chapter, walking in close community with others is paramount.[80]

Every day you must claim your freedom- and the remind yourself that you've done so. As Caroline Leaf writes, "The hardest part about achieving peak happiness, thinking, and health is remembering that we can choose them."[81]

Choose it. If you intend to experience it, you must intentionally decide to live free. **Freedom doesn't appear by accident. And you often experience it a season *after* you first claim it and begin fighting for it.**

That said, there is a tension here, something we've got to "own" about freedom and what it looks like. Many times when our bodies heal things go back to how they were. Not always, but often. A cut heals and the skin looks as good as new. A broken bone mends, often stronger than it ever was. Sometimes the wounds don't completely heal, though. A "new normal" happens. We walk with a limp or we still bear a scar. The same thing often occurs in life. Sometimes, the scars remain, even as we walk forward in freedom. In the next chapter we'll discuss how those scars often become the finest gold in our lives.

---

[80] I discuss this in detail at *Emotional Wholeness Checklist*.

[81] *Switch On Your Brain*, p139.

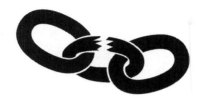

12. Gold in the Broken Places

I almost titled this chapter something like, *"What do you actually think restoration looks like?"*

I didn't, because it seemed a bit punchy for such a soft subject. But, after you read the next few pages, I think you'll understand that line from a place of tenderness. Perhaps even from a place of hope.

As we were going back and forth about the forward for this book, JB and I sat in a pub in downtown Salt Lake City discussing "hard things." He experienced his version of a few tough chapters just like me. Each of us have different details, and both stories were- *are*- difficult to live in their unique ways.

About the time the appetizers hit the table, JB observed, "Everyone looks at the book of Job as this great story of redemption."

"I used to," I confessed. "But I don't see it *just as that* anymore, though."

"Yeah, it's way more complex."

We discussed the tension between the beginning of the book (when Job's life is ripped right out from under him) and the end of the book (when things are "restored" multiple times over what he originally had). That's the *surface* read, anyway.

In the first few verses catastrophes rock him-

- Sabeans invade, taking his oxen and killing his servants (1:13).

- Fire falls from Heaven, obliterating his herd of sheep and the servants who tend them (1:16).

- Chaldeans scoop in, swiping his camels (1:17).

- Then, as if that's not enough, the big one: a strong wind breezes though, knocking the supports from beneath his home, causing the roof to fall and crush *all* of his kids, burying them alive (1:18-19).

His friends all blamed *him* for this. Surely, life wasn't working his way because of some secret clutter, a stashed away skeleton, or a pet sin he nurtured. That's what they told him (God later corrected them, by the way, attesting to Job's righteousness).

And, his wife *couldn't stand him*. She loathed the fact that he even breathed (19:17). She encouraged him to die. Yes, that's *exactly* how it's penned in the Bible.

"At the end of the story," JB said, "Job ends up with twice as much wealth as before. His net worth doubles overnight" (42:10). "In fact, the Bible says people actually brought money to Job, as an offering of love and support" (42:11).

"Yes," I said, "And he has seven more sons and three more daughters" (42:12).

"But, he still lost his family in the beginning. Restoration didn't mean they come back from the dead."

"And we have no idea what happened to his wife in all of this. We don't read much more about her. Did she stay around and see her way through it all? Or is it a different woman at the end of the story?"

We decided there's no way to know all of the answers to all of the questions this story raises. **We do know, though, that the restored life didn't look like a "cleaned up" and "returned" version of the old one.** He still mourned his kids for the rest of an extremely long life. He lost servants and co-workers who were once close to him. His friendships may never have been the same with the people who wrongfully accused him. Life was different.

"We lost Evans a few years ago," JB said. "We got through it. The Lord restored us. But my son is still dead. I still miss him. That's part of the tension."

In that moment I could sympathize. Not in the *same* way, but in *some* way. I spent a solid year jumping though every conceivable hoop and meeting every demand that was given to me. No matter how "good" I was or how hard I begged for relational healing, I was black-balled, ghosted, and met with legal shenanigans.

IT MAY NOT COME BACK

Restoration doesn't always mean return. We like to think that it does, but many times it doesn't.

I suppose I realized that about six months ago. I just didn't have language for it back then. That was about the time I really found myself grieving. I realized that things I hoped and prayed for would probably never return to the way they were.

The truth is that, after any difficult season, things may never return "just like they were before." And, in fact, if we're honest, we probably don't want them to be. Not "just like they were before," anyway.

It's easy to look back at life after a traumatic event (or events) and wish we could "just go back to how things used to be." **Our minds have a powerful way of not only causing us to avoid pain in the future (by perceiving reality in ways that protect us), but also by re-scripting the past such that we often remember a "greatest hits" or highlight reel rewind rather than the raw reality we endured.**

Because we often observe the rearview of life with rose-colored glasses, we tend to overlook some of the pain and dysfunction we've endured. When we take an honest assessment, we see it. And that means that, **even though no situation is perfect (nor ever will be), sometimes things *do* need to go back to "how it was" and sometimes they *don't*.**

For a season, one of the things that yanks us back to the past is grief, an extremely real emotion that we talk too little about.

- We experience grief that trauma came- and *pain happened*.

- Then we often feel grief over what *we expected* to happen next (perhaps an outcome, a redemption, a forgiveness withheld).

- There's grief over the *things we may miss in the future* (i.e., a spouse dies or abandons you, so it dawns on us that we won't celebrate future milestone anniversaries or grow old together, that our kids' weddings will not be laced with awkwardness and strange family dynamics rather than a unified front, etc.).

- There's grief over the notion *that we're even grieving*, and that we thought we'd be in a "different place" by this point in our lives.

It's all complex, and it's the stuff that needs to be sorted during those pauses of Sabbath and sleep. In other words, **grief and dealing with the hard things is one of the reasons we need to slow down and live in the right rhythm**.

THE WRONG SCALE

I want to highlight something that often- though not always- happens when people face situations that *demand* grief. Here it is: we often create a false scale of polar opposites. On one extreme, we place the label "imperfect" and on the other side "valuable." Any move towards the direction of imperfection by necessity pulls us farther away from valuable.

A FALSE SCALE

* WHEN WE FACE TOUGH SITUATIONS WE OFTEN WRONGLY CREATE A FALSE SCALE- THAT THINGS ARE EITHER PERFECT OR WE'RE WORTHLESS.

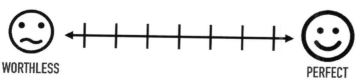

WORTHLESS   **PERFECT**

- THIS PROVES DESTRUCTIVE WHEN THEY PUT THEMSELVES ON THAT SCALE. B/C EVERYONE KNOWS THEY'RE NOT PERFECT!

Here's the result: The more *perfect* things are (including less "hard things," less emotional baggage, less spiritual clutter), the more *valuable* we perceive ourselves to be. The *worse* things are, the more *worthless* we perceive ourselves to be.

This is a difficult place to live- for several reasons:

- **First, most things in life are *clearly* out of our control.** Perfection- in any area- is *impossible*.

- **Second, the "worthless to perfect" scale is a false dichotomy anyway**. The opposite of *perfect* is imperfect- not worthless. And the opposite of worthless is *valuable*- not perfect.

TRUE OPPOSITES

THE OPPOSITE OF PERFECT IS "IMPERFECT"- NOT WORTHLESS.

IMPERFECT ←——|——|——|——|——|——→ **PERFECT**

THE OPPOSITE OF WORTHLESS IS "VALUABLE."

WORTHLESS ←——|——|——|——|——|——→ **VALUABLE**

In other words, it's possible to be imperfect and valuable at the same time. We can all agree that there are things we're great at, as well as things we're not so great at. In fact, this- *imperfect* and *valuable*- describes the human condition perfectly.

It's OK to affirm our value and simultaneously embrace the imperfections of life- even the ones which result from our poor decisions.

We often don't translate that message to their core identity, though. We often feel we deserve what we got... because we're not valuable.

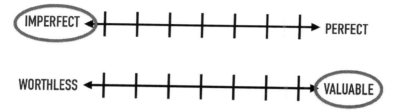

THE HUMAN CONDITION

IT'S POSSIBLE TO BE IMPERFECT AND VALUABLE AT THE SAME TIME! IT'S OK TO AFFIRM OUR VALUE AND EMBRACE OUR IMPERFECTION AT THE SAME TIME.

SOME SCARS REMAIN

I've spent the majority of my life in "church world." When you do that, you get to hear a lot of statements that sound right but just aren't true. Add to that today's propensity towards sound bites, memes, and tweet-able quotes and you've got a situation that's ripe for slick sounding *almost*-truths.

"Your wounds should never be part of your identity," some people say. "If they are, it shows you haven't fully healed yet."

Or, "You'll get over it."

Hogwash. Or whatever other phrase you want to throw in there.

A few years ago Jim Bob and Cindy lost a baby boy. After a rough few years, followed by a reconnection and restoration, Evans' birth seemed like redemption.

And then, within just a few hours, it didn't. He was gone.

Do you "get over" that?

"No," JB said. "But you do figure out a way to get *through* it. And **sometimes that means the scars remain. They no longer control the story, but they are part of it- perhaps even a significant part.**"

Let me back it with some Bible.

When they killed Jesus, they battered Him mercilessly. Isaiah prophesied the soldiers would beat Him so horrifically that you wouldn't be able to recognize who He was- or that He was even human (read Isaiah 53). They shredded His back, they forced a crown of thick thorns *into* (not just *onto*, but *into*) His skull, and they shoved a spear through His abdomen to puncture His heart.

After He arose from the dead, He bore *almost none* of those scars. That's right, *almost*.

Clearly, when the disciples questioned as to whether or not it was Him, He showed them certain scars which remained- the ones where the nails punctured Him and the wound on His side (John 20:20). In fact, *those* scars were His proof to a doubting Thomas that He was, indeed, Himself.

Jesus encouraged Thomas, "Look, see the wounds in My hands and on My side" (John 20:27).

I don't know the significance of some scars for some people as opposed to other scars for others. I do know, though, that some scars remain and others don't.

Perhaps part of the difference is that **whole people- those who've claimed their freedom and learned to walk with grace and health- don't *lead* with the scars**. Rather, they selectively, deliberately reveal them when those wounds can encourage, equip, and empower someone else to put one foot forward and begin their freedom march, too. That is, perhaps the sharing works best when it's no longer about the one who is now free, it's about those who remain in the struggle.

I don't know. I'm still processing it. I tend to write books for myself, about things I need to know, rather than things I've mastered. Right now, I'm trying to figure this one out...

I do know, though, that the narratives of our lives- the more whole we become- become a living version of *kintsukuroi,* Japanese art form in which broken pottery is repaired. Rather than restoring the piece to look as if it's never been damaged (which is, really, impossible), the artisan injects gold into the cracks as the pottery is restored.

The flaws are accentuated, celebrated. In other words, **not only are those flaws *not* hidden, they're actually highlighted.**

Yet, at the same time, **those scars never determine the shape of the vessel**. The identity originally given by its creator does.[82]

It's some what of an oxymoron, isn't it?

---

[82] Another example: Jacob became the Father of Israel. The nation is literally named after his second name, the one given to him by God. This happened after he wrestled with the angel all night, walking away with a permanent limp (see Genesis 32:22-32). There's a saying that goes "Never trust someone who doesn't walk with a limp." It's a nod to this event, that you can't trust someone who hasn't owned their flaws and then, in spite of them, clung to the Lord for His grace, His healing, and His blessing.

Google it. The "new" version of the pottery looks *like* the old, but better. It's simultaneously more raw and more beautiful than the original, untainted version.

Grace is the gold. And healing. And the wholeness we walk in as we *therapeuo* our way forward.

Furthermore, **the trifecta of grace + healing + wholeness means my imperfections now serve a greater purpose than the pain and shame originally created by them**. And the more golden those scars become, the more whole I am and the greater substance I can carry.

SIGNS OF SOMETHING BETTER

In the Old Testament we meet a prostitute named Rahab. Before taking over the Promised Land, Joshua sent two spies to scout the land. Apparently, they spent the night in her home. With all the "coming and going," they'd never be noticed. Plus, even if they were, no one would ever tattle about who was in the whore house with them. In doing so, they would rat themselves out.

She told those spies that the people in the of Jericho had been "melting in fear" of them for the previous 40 years (Joshua 2:11). Even though the Israelites were certain the "giants in the land" would smash *them*, the giants were the ones afraid (Numbers 13:33).

She told them, "Save me and my family."

The spies agreed- as long as she threw a red cord in the window of her home- the window that sat in the city wall (Joshua 2:18).

Where did the cord come from?

It came from her door. Before electricity made "red light districts" possible, scarlet cords were the signposts *prostitutes* and *madams* hung to denote they were open for business. She took that sign- the one thing that would have marked her as a woman of shame- and placed it in her window for the world to see. Everyone marching with Israel would see and know that the very thing which shamed her was now the thing that marked her for salvation (2:21). The red scar became gold.

Here's where things get even more interesting…

Not only is this woman mentioned in the Hall of Fame of Faith (Hebrews 11:31), but she's also an ancestor of King David. This makes her an ancestor of Jesus, the Author of and embodiment of the grace + healing + wholeness trio that creates that gold where the flaws once were. She's also listed in the genealogical records that we generally skip when we go looking for the Christmas story (Matthew 1:5).

And then there's this…

That red cord is featured all throughout the sacrificial system. Apparently, when the priest laid an offering on the altar, they also set a red cord atop it for everyone to see (Leviticus 14:49-51, Numbers 19:6).

"Let's just toss this skeleton that's in the closet right there into the middle of the room," the sacrificial system effectively communicates.

It's the ancient version of that Eminem rap from *8 Mile* we talked about in the intro.

How's that for irony?

Perhaps this is what Isaiah meant when he wrote, "Though your sins are like scarlet, they shall be as white as snow; though they are red like crimson, they shall become like wool" (1:18 ESV).[83]

Yes, grace works greatest when we strip the Accuser of his accusation, taking it and flipping it into a signifier of salvation.

GRACE IS RELATIONAL – NOT JUST INFORMATIONAL

Paul says we have a treasure in earthen vessels (2 Corinthians 4:7 TLV):

> … have have this treasure in jars of clay, so that the surpassing greatness of the power may be from God and not from ourselves.

We love that verse. We place it on coffee mugs and calendars and bookmarks.

Notice the next verses, though. They provide us with the context of the first (4:8-10 TLV):

> We are hard pressed in every way, yet not crushed; perplexed, yet not in despair; persecuted, yet not forsaken; struck down, yet not destroyed; always carrying in the body the death of [Jesus] so that the life of [Jesus] may also be revealed in our mortal body.

Notice the tension- the revelation shines in our flesh, in human form. **Jesus doesn't reveal Himself just through books; He reveals Himself through**

---

[83] Extra-canonical writings from the same time period report that after the sacrifices were offered, the cord mysteriously and supernaturally turned white. They also note that around 33AD, the time Christ was crucified, the cord stopped turning white. Why? Because the once-for-all sacrifice had been offered (see Hebrews 10:1f.).

the grit of the broken places. Through the gold that shines where the flaws once were.

Paul reminds us in *another* passage that it is precisely in the places in which he himself is weak that he- because of the presence of a living Christ that embodies him- becomes strong. Paul writes (2 Corinthians 12:10 NIV):

> *I delight in my weaknesses, in insults, in hardships, in persecutions, in difficulties. For when I am weak, then I am strong.*

I'm not there, yet- *delighting in the hard things*. But Paul is clear that God's power is made complete- *whole*- in the weak places (see 2 Corinthians 12:9). That is, He manifests in the fractures.

The gold can only be placed where there are cracks to be filled. No crack, no space. No space, no gold to fill the void. **Brokenness is the thing to which grace almost *exclusively* bonds**. As Donald Miller writes,

> *Grace only sticks to our imperfections. Those who can't accept their imperfections can't accept grace, either.*[84]

In recovery, you eventually get to Step 4, that infamous place where you pause and take a moral inventory of your life. I know firsthand. Not only have I written and shot film for a 12-step program, remember, I attended one.[85] Some of the stories in this book, in fact, are an overflow of my Step 4.

Sponsors tell you, "Don't just write down the bad. Step 4 an inventory of your life. Not just a list of your failures. It should be balanced."

I get it.

---

[84] *Scary Close*, page 45.

[85] Go to www.TheNextBestStep.info and download the course free of charge.

Yes, sometimes our stories may seem a bit lop-sided- slanted towards the bad. Especially when we're cleaning up the clutter and walking towards wholeness and freedom.

But that's where we meet grace. And it's where we truly uncover that grace is not a theological system or a random bit of verses strung together. Grace isn't even a sentimental feel that things are forgiven and *something* will work out for the best.

Sure, grace is that. All of it. But grace is more. Grace is a person. Grace has a name. Grace is called *Jesus*.

I avoided my story because there were things in it I couldn't fathom. Owning the story meant owning the main character of the story, me.

I've seen, though, that Jesus didn't come to condemn (John 3:17), He came to save. And He continues saving. Salvation is *now*.

During the New Testament era they were so certain that salvation was a now, in-this-lifetime experience that many of them punted off the promise of Heaven. Paul had to go out of this way and remind them that salvation is future, too.[86]

We often flip it backwards. We forget that Jesus invades life now. He always brings with him the fullness of grace (and truth) (see John 1:14). He moves us gently, graciously, from our past... to our potential.

And He does that completely... wounds, fractures, scars, and all. **He seals the cracks with the gold of grace so that we no longer leak our pain. Then He fills us... to the point that we overflow His presence.**

Kintsukuroi.

---

[86] Read 1 Corinthians 15, or listen to episode 18 of my podcast. There, I cover this idea in more detail.

May you be healed, may you walk in health, and may the gold in those scars highlight the possibility of wholeness to others. And **may you find peace not in the return of what *was*, but in a redemption to what *should be*.**

12. GOLD IN THE BROKEN PLACES

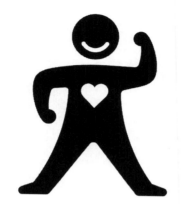

PART 2: THE OILS

PART 2: THE OILS

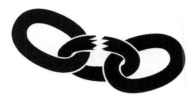

13. Freedom Sleep

The place to begin the "work" of handling tough emotional hurts is, oddly enough, sleep. We should pause before pushing forward into the hard work.[87]

There are a few reasons why:

- Sleep is when your body physically rebuilds (most people understand this), *as well as when your soul emotionally recovers* (many people don't grasp this).

- Sleep is when your mind, on its own, naturally sorts unfinished business from the waking hours, effectively "de-fragging" your mental mind like a computer de-frags its hard drive.

- Sleep is when your entire "system" powers down, allowing it to power up back in rhythm.

When we don't get enough rest, our bodies begin running on adrenaline. That makes it more difficult to wind down in the evening (thereby preventing us from

---

[87] Reviews chapters 7 & 8.

sleep) and it causes us to feel more zombie-like during the day (creating those mid-afternoon crashes).

Deliberate sleep is far different than "checking out" because you feel down or depressed (which are natural feelings, so don't shy away from those, either- they tell us something we need to know about what we're dealing with). Intentional sleep acknowledges that we're created to live in a rhythm of "off" and "on," and that emotional and mental recovery is just as important as physical rest. Taking time "off" is one of the best ways to live "on."

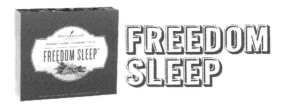

Young Living's Freedom Sleep (Item #4722) is the first of two essential oil kits in the Freedom Collection.

Aromatherapy works incredibly well as we step into this healthy rhythm of rest for several reasons:

- **Smell is the most powerful sense we have**, so we "work" from a position of strength when we tap into it.

- **Smell is tied to our survival instincts** (i.e., we avoid foods that smell spoiled, as well as things that are rotten or smell like trash- because the nose alerts us!). If you've endured a difficult season, your survival instincts have most likely been awakened.

- **Smell is tied to memory**, because of its association with the limbic system.[88] The smell of Fall leaves, certain baked goods, or even a perfume or cologne may conjure certain past memories, thereby "transporting" us to another time and place. With essential oils we can deal with harmful memories and seek wholeness and healing, because we leverage this power for health and wholeness.

This approach isn't new, by the way. In fact, "sacred" smells such as Frankincense and Sandalwood have been used for religious purposes for centuries. For instance, browse through the Old Testament and notice how often Frankincense appears (it's part of the anointing oil and the oil of incense).

The Freedom Sleep kit (Item #4722) includes four essential oil blends-

- Freedom

- Aroma Sleep

- Valor

- Inner Harmony

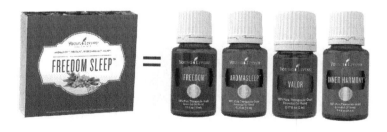

---

[88] I won't go into the limbic system in this book. We've discussed it in more detail in our books Health + Healing & Essential Oils (about the Oils of Ancient Scripture) and Essential Oils 101. Go to www.OilyApp.com/books to access the online courses or for links to purchase the paperback books.

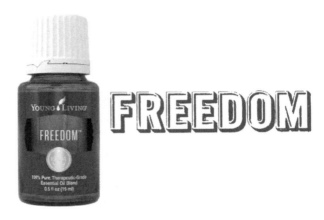

The oil: *Freedom*

What's in it: Some of the oils in this blend include Sacred Frankincense, Vetiver, Lavender, Idaho Blue Spruce, Peppermint, Palo Santo, Valerian, and Rue.

- Palo Santo was used by the Incas to cleanse the air of negative energies, as well as for good luck.

Known for: Freedom encourages a positive energy flow throughout the body and enhances the other oils in the Freedom Sleep kit. Whereas you can use the alone with great effectiveness, it amplifies the others when used in combination with them.

Freedom helps you identify the negative emotions and begin the healing process. It is the starting point.

How to apply it: Place 2 drops on the soles of your feet as you prepare to go to bed.

Note: this oil is included in both the Freedom Sleep kit and Freedom Release kit.

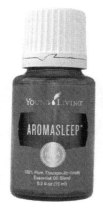

The oil: *Aroma Sleep*

What's in it: Lavender, Geranium, Bergamot, Valerian, and Sacred Frankincense are significant ingredients of this blend.

- Lavender is highly regarded for its soothing properties, immediately evoking a sense of peace.

- Geranium "helps release negative memories and eases nervous tension. It balances the emotions, lifts the spirit, and fosters peace, well-being, and hope."[89]

Known for: Aroma Sleep is calming, relaxing, and balancing- *physically and emotionally.* Remember, sleep is not only when your body recovers, it's also when your mind rejuvenates and your emotions reset. Aroma Sleep works with your brain to slow down, pause, and move towards rest.

How to apply it: 2 drops on the back of the neck.

---

[89] Source: *Essential Oil Pocket Reference*

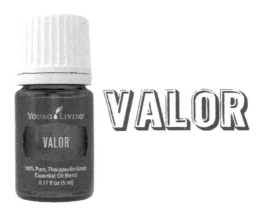

The oil: *Valor*

What's in it: Black Spruce, Blue Tansy, Camphor, and Geranium are constituents.

- Black Spruce "releases emotional blocks," as well as "brings feelings of balance and grounding."[90]

- Blue Tansy gives Valor it's distinctive purple-blue color.

Known for: Valor encourages a feeling of self control and helps overcome anger and negative emotions. Many times, traumatic events cause us to feel angry and fearful at the same time. In fact, we may feel a complex cocktail of emotions that are difficult to sort. Valor helps us "pull it together."

Known as "courage in a bottle," Valor empowers us to acknowledge the hard things and step forward anyway. Many times, the hardest thing is pressing the pause button, closing your eyes, and letting life go on while you take a restorative break.

How to apply it: 2 drops on the chest and heart as you prepare for bed.

---

[90] Source: *Essential Oil Pocket Reference*

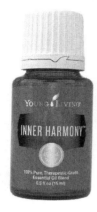

INNER HARMONY

The oil: *Inner Harmony*

What's in it: Geranium, Lavender, Royal Hawaiian Sandalwood, Ylang Ylang, Idaho Blue Spruce, Sacred Frankincense, Northern Lights Black Spruce, Rose, and Myrrh are all in Inner Harmony.

- Ylang Ylang is noted for easing cardiac tension as well as feelings of depression. It also "combats anger, combats low self esteem, increases focus of thoughts, filters out negative energy, restores confidence and peace..."[91] Ylang Ylang is also a natural aphrodisiac (this might be important, as sex generally tapers during hard seasons, yet it's a natural stress release).

Known for: Inner Harmony helps release negative memories, calms the mind, and fosters peace. The blend helps you let go of the chaos, gather your thoughts, and pull your feelings together in alignment.

How to apply it: 2 drops on the wrists.

---

[91] Source: *Essential Oil Pocket Reference*

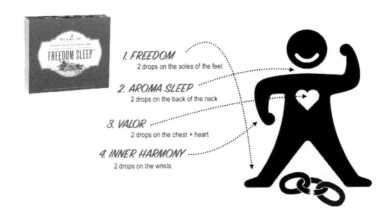

1. FREEDOM
2 drops on the soles of the feet

2. AROMA SLEEP
2 drops on the back of the neck

3. VALOR
2 drops on the chest + heart

4. INNER HARMONY
2 drops on the wrists

The Freedom Sleep kit (Item #4722) is designed for-

- Anyone suffering from negative life experiences

- People wanting the rejuvenating effects of going to bed more relaxed[92]

We suggest you create a nightly routine whereby you enjoy a 10-15 minute "night time ritual" that might involve brushing your teeth, setting your diffuser in your bedroom, and then applying each oil as you sit on the side of your bed.[93]

Make sure there are no "screens" or devices nearby, as the lights mitigate against sleep- and, any social feeds or emails you receive might evoke a response before you try to rest.

---

[92] In other words, even if you don't feel like you've endured something traumatic yet still have trouble sleeping, the kit may work for you. Sometimes we become so accustomed to going "full throttle" so long that we forget how to slow down. We become used to the work load.

[93] Suggestion for the diffuser: Use a different oil each night (2-3 drops) until you determine which you like best. Or, you may want to use something readily available (and more economical) like Lavender or Peace & Calming, allowing you to save your Freedom Sleep oils for topical use.

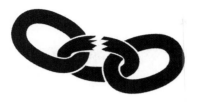

14. Freedom Release

The second kit in the Freedom Collection is Freedom Release (Item #4734), a collection of oils designed to help you not only rest and recover from hard things (the necessary first step) but resurrect and rebuild after enduring them (the second, *also necessary*, step if you're going to move forward and not find yourself stuck in the past).

The two kits are designed to enhance one another and be used as a whole.

We'll discuss the oils in the Freedom Release kit (Item #4734), as well as how to apply them. Then, we'll outline ways in which you can use these kits together in order to attain the maximum benefits of both.

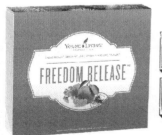

The Freedom Release kit (Item #4734) is perfect for-

- Anyone suffering from negative life experiences

- People wanting to release frustration, anger, and depression

- Those seeking emotional balance, positive energy flow, and a hopeful outlook on life

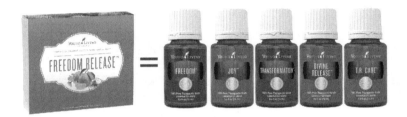

The Freedom Release kit (Item #4734) includes five essential oil blends-

- Freedom (part of both Freedom Sleep & Freedom Release)

- Joy

- Transformation

- Divine Release

- T.R. Care

Whereas you use the Freedom Sleep kit in the evening, you'll use the Freedom Release kit in the morning.

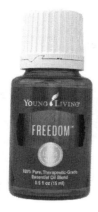

FREEDOM

The oil: *Freedom* (part of both kits)

What's in it: Some of the oils in this blend include Sacred Frankincense, Vetiver, Lavender, Idaho Blue Spruce, Peppermint, Palo Santo, Valerian, and Rue.

- When we discussed the Freedom blend as part of the Sleep kit we mentioned Palo Santo. Here, we'll highlight Valerian. Valerian is known around the world as an anti-insomnia plant. As well, "during the past three decades, Valerian has been clinically investigated for its tranquilizing effects on the central nervous system."[94] The plant is said to ease restlessness and calm tension, allowing you to face your day.

Known for: Freedom encourages a positive energy flow throughout the body.

How to apply it: Place 2 drops on the soles of your feet, ready to move forward.

---

[94] Source: *Essential Oil Pocket Reference*

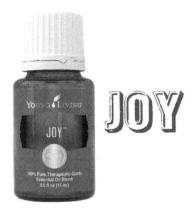

The oil: *Joy*

What's in it: Bergmot, Ylang Ylang, Geranium, Lemon, Tangerine, Jasmine, and Rose are all found in Joy.

- Bergamot is believed to have been taken by Christopher Columbus from the Canary Islands to Bergamo, Italy. It has a calming effect, and it's a strong hormonal support (hormones are involved with the endocrine system, which manages stress).[95] People in Columbus' day who sailed and explored for years at a time, thereby becoming homesick, believed Bergamot was an antidepressant for weary travelers who still needed to "show up" for their day.

Known for: Joy helps cope with grief and helps relax & calm the mind, provoking a sense of wellbeing.

How to apply it: 2 drops on the heart.

---

[95] Learn more about this in our online course at https://www.oilyapp.com/stressshield (case-sensitive, all lowercase).

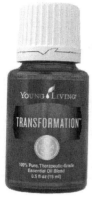

TRANSFORMATION

The oil: *Transformation*

What's in it: Lemon, Peppermint, Royal Hawaiian Sandalwood, Sacred Frankincense, Idaho Blue Spruce, Ocotea, and Palo Santo comprise this blend.

- Ocotea promotes "feelings of fullness." It's also said to release hypertension and anxiety, as well as provide digestive support (a wonky stomach often accompanies stressful seasons).

Known for: Transformation helps unlock repressed memories from the deep recesses of the mind. It stimulates a "positive reversal" of outlook, so that you might move forward.

Transformation may help you write new neuro-pathways as you heal from old memories and build new ones.[96] It works with your body to bring up the old, let it go, and renovate the soul.

How to apply it: 2 drops on your wrists, at the pulse points.

---

[96] For more on "neuro-plasticity," see Elizabeth Erickson's book, *Mind Your Brain*.

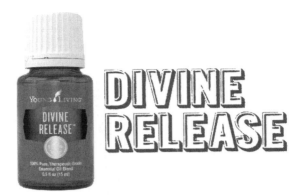

The oil: *Divine Release*

What's in it: Angelica, Rose, and Helichrysum, among others. Two highlights-

- Rose is a relaxant which "helps bring balance and harmony, allows one to overcome insecurities," that is, a feeling often associated with people who've survived hard things.[97]

- Angelica was historically referred to as the "Holy Spirit Root" and "Oil of the Angels," because of its healing properties. It was believed to supernaturally protect people from plagues. For our purposes, it "assists in the release of pent-up negative feelings and restores memories to... before trauma was ever perceived."[98]

Known for: Releasing anger. Benjamin Franklin said it best, "To err is human..." (Right? Everyone messes up.) And, "To forgive... is divine."

How to apply it: 2 drops on the temples or crown chakra.

---

[97] Source: *Essential Oil Pocket Reference*

[98] Source: *Essential Oil Pocket Reference*

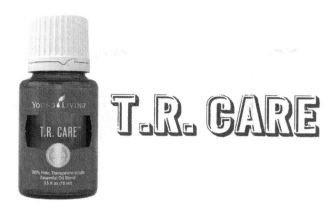

The oil: *T.R. Care* (often referred to as *Trauma Release Care*)

What's in it: Constituents include Roman Chamomile, Lavender, Bergamot, Frankincense, Valerian, Blue Cypress, Royal Hawaiian Sandalwood, & Cedarwood.

- Roman Chamomile "minimizes anxiety, irritability, and nervousness." Further, it helps "stabilize the emotions" and "helps release emotions that are linked to the past."[99]

Known for: Replacing emotions. The old ones must be replaced with something positive or they return. T.R. Care helps us step forward, rebuilding as we go.

How to apply it: Apply 2 drops to the edge of the ears.[100] Notably, in the Old Testament, this is how the priests and lepers were anointed as one group was tapped to serve the community of faith and the other was restored back into it.

---

[99] Source: *Essential Oil Pocket Reference*

[100] Auriculotherapy (also auricular therapy, ear acupuncture, and auriculoacupuncture) is a form of alternative medicine based on the idea that the ear is a micro system, which reflects the entire body, represented on the auricle, the outer portion of the ear. Conditions affecting the physical, mental or emotional health of the patient are assumed to be treatable by stimulation of the surface of the ear exclusively.(https://en.wikipedia.org/wiki/Auriculotherapy)

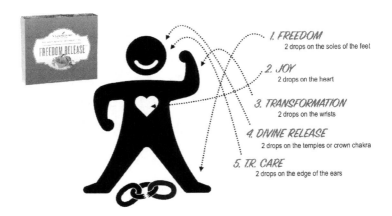

1. FREEDOM
2 drops on the soles of the feet

2. JOY
2 drops on the heart

3. TRANSFORMATION
2 drops on the wrists

4. DIVINE RELEASE
2 drops on the temples or crown chakra

5. T.R. CARE
2 drops on the edge of the ears

Notice how the oils in the Freedom Release kit work together:

- *Freedom* prepares our emotional centers.

- We overcome grief with *Joy*.

- *Transformation* empowers us to adjust our thinking patterns and embrace a new outlook.

- *Divine Release* equips us to eliminate un-grace, un-forgiveness, and bitterness.[101]

- *T.R. Care* then encourages us to continue rebuilding, recognizing that our best self isn't just about overcoming the past, it's about living to our full potential.

---

[101] Yes, forgiveness, letting go of the past, is the very nature of the Creator and Redeemer. Since we're made in His image, we're not designed to hold un-grace, un-forgiveness or bitterness in our heart. Each one erodes the soul.

Days 1-30   Days 31-60

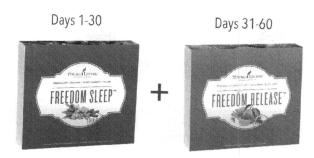

The Freedom Release kit (Item #4734) is a companion kit for the Freedom Sleep kit (Item #4722). Both products work so well together, that Young Living suggests you use them a single unit.

First, you rest. Use the Freedom Sleep kit for 30 days. Allow your body to rejuvenate and rebuild, recognizing that rest is some of the most important work you can do.

Second, rebuild. Use the Freedom Release kit for the next 30 days. After resting, you're ready to do the next phase of the "tough work" or resurrecting and recreating yourself.

Some people choose to use their kits together for days 31-60, opting to use the Freedom Release kit in the morning as they prepare to face their day and maintaining their evening rhythm of using the Freedom Sleep kit as they prepare to sleep.

Others choose to alternative, using the each kit for 30 days at a time.

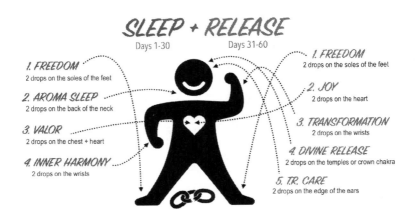

SLEEP + RELEASE

Days 1-30   Days 31-60

1. FREEDOM
2 drops on the soles of the feet

2. AROMA SLEEP
2 drops on the back of the neck

3. VALOR
2 drops on the chest + heart

4. INNER HARMONY
2 drops on the wrists

1. FREEDOM
2 drops on the soles of the feet

2. JOY
2 drops on the heart

3. TRANSFORMATION
2 drops on the wrists

4. DIVINE RELEASE
2 drops on the temples or crown chakra

5. T.R. CARE
2 drops on the edge of the ears

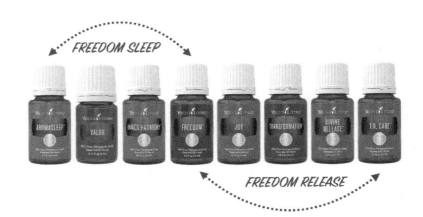

FREEDOM SLEEP

FREEDOM RELEASE

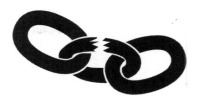

15. OOS Alternatives

The Freedom kits stay in high demand and regularly go out of stock (OOS) as soon as they are offered. For this reason, I recommend that you purchase the kits whenever they become available (even if you don't think you need them at that time) and that you maintain a supply of alternative oils when when they are not.

Since most the oils in the kits are only available as part of the kit(s) and are not offered on their own, you'll need to make substitutions. Here's what to substitute.

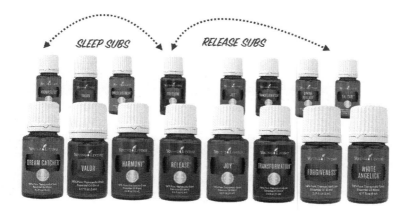

SLEEP SUBSTITUTIONS

For both kits, I suggest using Release in place of Freedom.

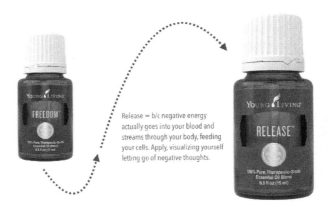

Release = b/c negative energy actually goes into your blood and streams through your body, feeding your cells. Apply, visualizing yourself letting go of negative thoughts.

In addition to purchasing Release instead of Freedom, you'll need to make two others swaps. Valor is the only oil from this kit that can be bought apart from the kit.

- Freedom = Release (Item #3408)

- Aroma Sleep = There are three options here. Choose Dream Catcher (#3330), Tranquil roll-on (Item #3533), or Rutavala oil (#3419) or Rutavala roll-on (#4471).

- Valor = this blend stays in stock and can be ordered on its own (Item #3430); also consider the roll-on option (#3529)

- Inner Harmony = Harmony (#3351)

There are several options for the Aroma Sleep substitution, but I've pictured Dream Catcher, my first choice.

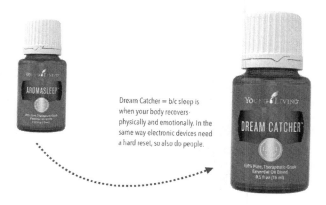

Dream Catcher = b/c sleep is when your body recovers - physically and emotionally. In the same way electronic devices need a hard reset, so also do people.

Harmony is a close counter-part to Inner Harmony, making it a logical sub.

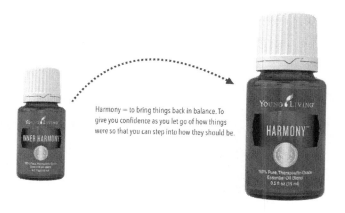

Harmony = to bring things back in balance. To give you confidence as you let go of how things were so that you can step into how they should be.

RELEASE SUBSTITUTIONS

To "build your own" Release kit, again, begin by using Release in place of Freedom. Joy and Transformation can both be purchased as stand-alones.

Here's the point-by-point list:

- Freedom = Release (Item #3408)

- Joy = this blend stays in stock and can be ordered on its own (Item #3372)

- Transformation = this blend stays in stock and can be ordered on its own (Item #3060)

- Divine Release = Forgiveness (#3339) or Surrender (Item #3424)

- T.R. Care = White Angelica (Item #3428) or Awaken (Item #3349)

For Divine Release I've provided you with two options. My first recommendation is Forgiveness. Surrender is another oil that may be selected as an alternative.

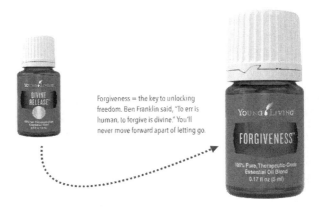

Forgiveness = the key to unlocking freedom. Ben Franklin said, "To err is human, to forgive is divine." You'll never move forward apart of letting go.

Since T.R. Care is only available through the kit, I suggest purchasing White Angelica in its place.

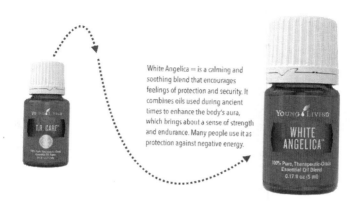

White Angelica = is a calming and soothing blend that encourages feelings of protection and security. It combines oils used during ancient times to enhance the body's aura, which brings about a sense of strength and endurance. Many people use it as protection against negative energy.

SUGGESTED KIT SWAP +

Four of the oils listed above as suggested substitutions are available in the Feelings Kit (#3125). The kit includes Release (sub for Freedom), Valor, Harmony (sub for Inner Harmony), Forgiveness (sub for Divine Release), meaning you could purchase:

- Feelings Kit

- Dream Catcher (or another alternative for Aroma Sleep)

- Joy

- Transformation

- White Angelica or Awaken as an alternative to T.R. Care

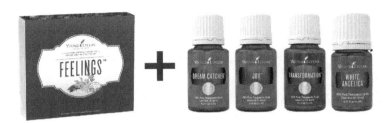

Taking this approach will leave you with 8 oils needed for your Freedom kits, as well as the additional oils from the Feelings Kit (Present Time and Inner Child). I wrote extensively about the Feelings Kit in the book *Emotional Wholeness Checklist.*

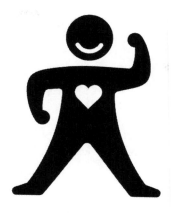

PART 3: BONUS MATERIALS

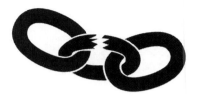

16. The Cost Issue

The Freedom Sleep kit (Item #4722) and Freedom Release kit (Item #4734) are two of the more costly kits in Young Living's inventory. Even at that, they're in constant demand and regularly go out of stock once inventory is replenished.

I suggest you purchase both kits at the same time, whenever they become available.

People regularly ask me about the cost. Generally, the follow-up question isn't meant to demean the money, but it's a genuine, "Is it worth it?" And "Does it work?" type of questioning.

First, yes, it's worth it. Here's why: *you're worth it.*

Throughout this book I've talked freely about spending money on counseling, therapy, a psychological evaluation, and other means to walk in mental and emotional health. These are all investments *in my soul*.

I believe that it's time we, as a culture, value our soul-wholeness as much as we value our physical fitness. Both matter.

I saw a meme floating around social media a few days ago that says much the same thing. Comparing how we spend the same dollar amounts on different items, it ready something like-

Healthy groceries ($100) = "too expensive"

Dinner date ($100) = "reasonable"

Therapist ($130) = "absurd"

Trip to Target ($130) = "great deals!"

Average college class ($1,000) = "expensive"

iPhone ($1,000) = "a necessity"

Kid's summer camp ($180) = "too much"

New pair of shoes ($180) = "they were on sale"

60 minutes of exercise = "I wish I had time!"

60 minutes on Instagram = "OMG time flies!"

1 hour on the phone with parents = "eternity"

1 hour watching Netflix = "let's watch another one"

The text-laden graphic concluded, "Everything in life is about priorities."

The obvious conclusion was simply this: *What do you value?*

Second, people ask me if it works. My reply is always something like "it works *if you work it.*"

Oils alone won't "fix" anyone. They're not designed to. But, they are a vital component of walking in *therapeuo*- that kind of health we discussed in chapter 11.

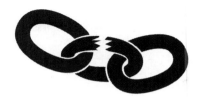

17. Redemption = Freedom

NOTE: I PLACED THIS CHAPTER HERE, AS IT PROVIDES THE BASIS FOR MOST OF THE CONCEPTS I TEACH.

I used to believe emotional health was just a "pop psychology" thing (which may, in part, explain how my own spirituality masked so much emotional dysfunction). I grew up *not* trusting what people- *including myself-* felt. On the other hand, I *trusted* what I read in the Bible.

Then I learned something profound. This has *everything* to do with inner healing, and the reality that it can- and does- happen. In fact, in my opinion, this chapter may be the most important one in the book because it provides you with the foundational cause of all soul healing.

Peter, one of Jesus' disciples, writes that we are redeemed by the blood of Jesus (1 Peter 1:18-19). *Redemption* is a common "Bible word," a term we read a lot and say a great deal- but one of those we don't really understand.

The word *redemption* was in common use in the ancient world. Specifically, the word *redemption* "was used in slave markets to refer to the price paid either to purchase a person, or to purchase that person's release."[102]

Outside of the church today, we see the word used in pawn shops. When someone comes to "free" their property which has been held; they pay the *redemption price* and their property is loosed to them.[103] (You're probably beginning to make theological connections even now.)

THE LAW OF FIRST MENTION

In seminary I learned about "the law of first mention," a precept that tells us to really comprehend something in the Biblical narrative, we need to dig deep into the first time we see the word or concept introduced. To understand *redemption* and the redeeming work of Jesus, and to comprehend everything achieved by His blood, we need to travel way back through the Old Testament to the book Exodus. The story of Israel's freedom provides incredible insight into the life Jesus offers each of us.

The first time we see the word *redemption* used is in Exodus 6:6- when the Lord mentions that He *will redeem* His people.

---

102 Mahesh Chavda, *The Hidden Power of the Blood of Jesus*, page 76.

103 Mary K. Baxter, *The Power of the Blood*, page 128.

God tells Moses to tell all of Israel, "I *will deliver you from slavery*... I will *redeem* you with an outstretched arm and with great acts of judgment" (6:6 ESV, emphasis added).

God refers to *redemption* in the future tense. It's not yet happened.

This is the word He declared for Moses to communicate to the people: "You will be free!" That's what God meant by redemption: *freedom*.

Or, to say it another way, "You're destined for redemption!"

Or, like the title of this book reads, "Claim your freedom."

To repeat, the first time we see the word appear is when God is telling His people, "I will redeem- *free*- you from slavery!" He says that redemption is a *future* thing He will do.

The second time we see the word *redeem* used in the Bible is in Exodus 15:13 when Miriam begins singing *after* the Children of Israel walk through the Red Sea. She celebrates, "These are the people whom You *have* redeemed." Whereas Moses heard about redemption as a future action, Miriam refers to it as something that's just occurred.

Notice it:

- The first use of *redeem* promises that God will free His people (Exodus 6:6)

- The second use of *redeem* declares that God has done it (Exodus 15:13)

- The only event in between the two usages is the the Exodus- the word *redeem* is used to describe

Clearly, the word points to the Exodus- to *God's deliverance of His people from slavery.*

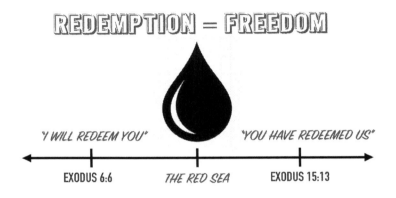

Fast forward another fourteen hundred years or so...

When Jesus is born, we're told that He is the Redeemer. That is, He is the One who brings freedom from slavery. *Redemption* is a word that links Jesus to freedom- to a freedom from the yoke of bondage. *Redemption* means "freedom." And it means freedom *now*, not later.

Looking *back* at the life of Christ (in the same way Miriam looked back at the Exodus), Paul reminds the leaders of the Church at Ephesus that Jesus *redeemed* the church by His blood (Acts 20:22).[104] In other words, because of what He achieved, something is now *different*. History has *changed*. Our destiny has been *altered*. We've been *transformed*.

---

[104] In the same way Miriam looks at God's people walking through the Red Sea, Paul looks at God's people walking in triumphant procession (2 Corinthians 2:14).

Revelation 5:9-10 contains the lyrics a song being offered to Jesus, stating one of the key reasons He is worthy of worship- namely, He *redeemed* us. The saints all sing in one accord: "You were slain, and You have *redeemed* us to God by your blood."

Notice the final phrase of the previous verse: "by your blood." It's the blood that redeems; it's the blood that sets us free.

TOTAL FREEDOM = BETTER THAN YOU WERE TAUGHT

Remember the verse we referenced from Peter?

He wrote, "You were not redeemed with corruptible things, like silver or gold, from your aimless conduct received by tradition from your fathers, but with the precious blood of [Jesus] Christ, as a lamb without blemish and spot" (1 Peter 1:18-19).[105]

Notice:

- We were redeemed (read: freed), by

- The precious blood of Jesus

Since we've been redeemed (freed), let's discover each of the following:

- What does Jesus redeem us from?

---

[105] Recall, these are similar to the lyrics to the song which the saints sing in Heaven, which we just read a few pages ago (Revelation 5:9-10).

- Where did Jesus achieve the work of redemption?

- What does Jesus redeem us to?

What are we redeemed from?

Most often, people answer with something like this: "Sin. Jesus redeems us from sin."

The writers of the New Testament go farther, however. Jesus redeems us from sin- and so much more. In the same way that God didn't redeem Israel from slavery to simply let them linger in the wilderness, Jesus doesn't just redeem us from the bad, He redeems us to our destiny.[106]

(I know. That's a lot of background info. I promise you… this is going somewhere.)

About the third or fourth time reading the Gospels and comparing each writer's interpretation of the Cross to the Exodus event, I caught it: Jesus' sacrifice at the Cross did far more than I had imagined.[107]

Here's one of the factors that helped me "see" it…

One of the authors I was reading side-by-side with the Scripture posed what *seemed* like a simple question: "*Where* did Jesus redeem us…?"

The obvious answer was this: "At the Cross." That's what I was studying, *the Cross.* That's what I was reading about. That's the centerpiece of the Christian faith. It's the

---

[106] Furthermore, like the Children of Israel, *we are redeemed to God.* We are not merely freed *from* bondage- we are freed *to* the Lord. This such an important idea (not only being freed *from* something but being freed *to* something) that we'll continue circling back to it. Remember, Jesus Himself was adamant that the one whom He sets free is "free indeed" (see John 8:36). In saying this He emphasized the certainly of the freedom.

[107] See *Redemption*, page 69.

event that changed all of history, right? "The Cross" is *always* the right answer, right?

The authors of several books I was reading at that time suggested that Jesus didn't *just* redeem us at the Cross, though. I know. Bold statement.

Here's the line of reasoning:

- First, the Bible says that we were redeemed by His blood (i.e., 1 Peter 1:18-19, Revelation 5:9, etc.). Most Christians aren't surprised to hear this. We've heard it for as long as we've been around the Church.

- Second, since Jesus redeemed us by His blood, it makes sense that He redeemed us *at each place He shed His blood.*[108]

Pause.

Rewind and review the second point. The place Jesus bled is important. That is, how and where Jesus bled actually reveals something as to the freedom(s) He grants us.

Peter says that we are redeemed *by the blood of Jesus* (1 Peter 1:18-19). He doesn't say that we are redeemed "at the Cross." Yes, it's easy to just *assume* that he's taking about the Cross. But, when we read the text we see something greater happening.

We are redeemed by the blood that Jesus shed at the Cross- *and during the events surrounding the Cross.* Peter emphasizes the blood, not necessary the location of the blood.

---

[108] See Larry Huch's book, *The Seven Places Jesus Shed His Blood.*

Think about the blood of Jesus for a moment, and all of the places we see it in the Bible. He bled in *seven* unique places.

1. In the Garden, He prayed and sweat great drops of blood.

2. As they soldiers came and arrested Him, they beat Him ruthlessly and He bled more, becoming bruised and battered even beyond recognition.

3. The Roman soldiers scourged Him, opening most of His back, exposing His internal organs... and His blood.

4. They mocked Him by placing a crown of thorns on his brow, causing more blood to flow.

5. They nailed His hands into the cross-beam, and He bled.

6. His feet became another place of bleeding.

7. Even after Jesus was confirmed to dead, a soldier pierced His side, puncturing His heart and releasing more blood.

Jesus literally shed *all* of His blood- *all of His blood for all of your redemption.*

This doesn't minimize the work of the Cross at all. Rather, it *amplifies* it. Understanding the full scope of what Jesus did for us is like plugging the victory declared from the Cross into an amplifier. Jesus bled at (at least) seven distinct places- not just one- and each place brought another degree of redemption with it.

Notice the chart on the following page.

WHERE & HOW JESUS BLED

WHERE IT HAPPENED	PLACE HE BLED	BIBLICAL REFERENCE
In the Garden	Sweat blood	Luke 22:44
Beaten in the Garden...	Bruising	Luke 22:64, Isaiah 53:5, 50:6
At the Roman palace	His back, scourging	Matthew 27:26, Mark 15:15
In the Roman Praetorium	Crown of thorns	Matthew 27:29, Mark 15:16
On the Cross	His hands	Matthew 27:35, Mark 15:24, Luke 23:33, John 19:18
On the Cross	His feet	Matthew 27:35, Mark 15:24, Luke 23:33, John 19:18
The Cross- after dying	Pierced heart	John 19:31-34

WHAT IT MEANS = TOTAL FREEDOM

Numerous theologians point to Jesus' back- referenced in Isaiah 53:5- and remind us that when He bled from his back He healed our physical bodies ("By His stripes you are healed."). Others suggest the blood from the crown of thorns reverses the curse of the thorns in Genesis 3. Jesus redeems the work of our hands, giving us back dominion and authority. I could go on- and I do in my book *Redemption*.[109]

---

[109] Download it free on my website or purchase it on Amazon. Go to www.Jenkins.tv/Redemption for more info.

For the purposes of mental and emotional healing, which is our topic here, let's look at two of the specific places Jesus bled.

First, Jesus was bruised.

Isaiah declared, "He was *wounded* for our transgressions; He was *bruised* for our iniquities" (53:5, emphasis added). Most translators agree that wounds and bruises are two different facets of healing:

- *Wounds* = external hurts

- *Bruises* = internal hurts

That is, Jesus heals our bodies (physical healing) and he heals... *bruises*?

A bruise happens when blood vessels burst beneath the skin, creating internal bleeding. Though visible from the outside, a bruise is an inside injury.

Make note, then, Jesus bled to heal the junk inside of us. That is, He didn't just died to forgive our sins and take our guilt, He also died to heal the mental and emotional clutter that accompanies sin- the sins we commit and the sins committed against us.

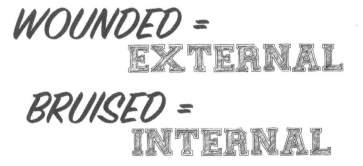

WOUNDED = EXTERNAL
BRUISED = INTERNAL

Sin isn't just an action that's "done" and then gone. Sin often leads a wound, a mark, and an uncleanness that attaches itself to the soul. It's *internal*.

Physical bruises can become so much a part of our outside appearance that you may not have even made the correlation that bruises are actually blood vessels which have burst beneath the skin. Our "internal" wounds and emotional hurts are the same, right? If we don't deal with them in a healthy way, even though we try desperately to hide them, our emotional wounds become visible to everyone around us in an unhealthy way.

In fact, these internal wounds can become the filter whereby we begin interpreting the world around us. You see it in my story-

- When I was a kid, I performed religious routines, putting myself on a performance scale, because of the rejection I felt when I was younger- and all as the applause I received for doing well.

- I continued living on a performance scale, placing my value in what I did rather than who I am. This caused me to plow over anyone who stood in my way, seeing them as a barrier to my success. It even caused me to see a "needy" wife and "demanding" children as hindrances to success rather than blessings to be enjoyed.

- I had a difficult time letting people "up close" because of so many times I was rejected when I was younger. That became a bruise that became part of my identity.

We can become so accustomed to these bruises that we hardly notice them. Though obvious to those around us, we're often blind to some of the very hurts which cause many of our ongoing struggles. They become our perceptions, our default mode of interpreting the world around us (and, remember, perception isn't always reality- sometimes, we get it wrong).

Furthermore, you've been hurt enough- or seen people who've hurt enough- to see that if you don't resolve the emotional wound, the bruise becomes larger and larger, causing more and more issues...

Let's get personal about this. If you identify yourself based on the past, *the wound has marked you*. The bruise, though "beneath the surface," is probably visible to everyone around you. It's become part of your identity, and may even be your most predominant feature- just like my emotional dysfunction had become.

Walking with a bruise is every different than living with a scar. A bruise remains tender. A scar, by its very nature, verifies that healing has happened or is, at least, significantly underway.

When Jesus bled beneath His skin, He redeemed / freed everything in side us.

STILL WORKING FOR YOU

Second, there's another place Jesus bled I want to highlight to you, though, another places that has to deal with emotional healing...

Grasp this: **Jesus' work on the Cross is so thorough that even *after* Jesus died He continued bleeding**. This is important to note, because "the wages of sin is death" (Romans 3:23). All that was really *required* for our forgiveness was that a sacrifice be made for sins.

On the Cross, Jesus declared "It is finished" (John 19:30). Then, He committed His Spirit to the Father and died (Luke 23:46). At this point, *sin had been atoned for.*

Even after all things are complete, though, Jesus did more. *Additional redemption was offered*

We read in the Gospels that Jesus bled even *after* He died, even *after* sin was handled. Since we know that every place Jesus bled He redeemed something for us, we know that- even after His death- He still claimed more freedom for us!

John is the only writer to pen the following detail (see John 19:31-34). He writes that after Jesus died "one of the soldiers pierced His side with a spear, and immediately blood and water came out" (19:34).

What was He doing?

Why continue bleeding after He was dead?

Wasn't He done?

I mean, He said it was finished, right?

From the outset of His ministry, Jesus proclaimed that He came to bind the broken-hearted (Luke 4:18). Since we know we can trust His word, we can assume He heals those who have emotional hurts. When John declares that Jesus bled from His heart, He shows us the actual time and place where Jesus purchased this freedom for us.

The more I dive into the depth of what Jesus achieved for us- and what He continues to do in us- the more I see that:

- He's not overwhelmed by the number of wounds we have

- He's not offended at us for the damage we've inflicted in ourselves

- He never ostracizes us for the hurt we've caused others

REDEMPTION OF THE SOUL = THE LEFT SIDE

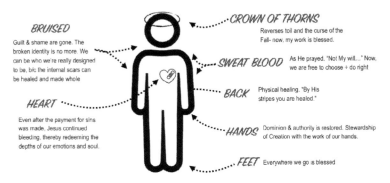

BRUISED

Guilt & shame are gone. The broken identity is no more. We can be who we're really designed to be, b/c the internal scars can be healed and made whole

HEART

Even after the payment for sins was made, Jesus continued bleeding, thereby redeeming the depths of our emotions and soul.

CROWN OF THORNS

Reverses toil and the curse of the Fall- now, my work is blessed.

SWEAT BLOOD As He prayed, "Not My will..." Now, we are free to choose + do right

BACK Physical healing. "By His stripes you are healed."

HANDS Dominion & authority is restored. Stewardship of Creation with the work of our hands.

FEET Everywhere we go is blessed

The promise of total redemption has no expiration date, no exclusion clauses, and no ineligible recipients.

Your freedom has been paid for.

It's time to claim it. All of it.

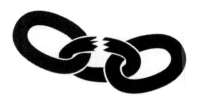

18. Self-Evaluation / Post Traumatic Stress Test

THE FOLLOWING SELF-EXAMINATION IS PROVIDED FOR PERSONAL EXPLORATION ONLY. IT IS NOT INTENDED TO DIAGNOSE, TREAT, OR PRESCRIBE. IF YOU FEEL LIKE YOU NEED HELP, YOU SHOULD CONSULT THE CARE OF A LICENSED PROFESSIONAL.

NOTE: THE PTSD SELF-CHECK IS ALSO AVAILABLE ONLINE AT JENKINS.TV/PTSD.

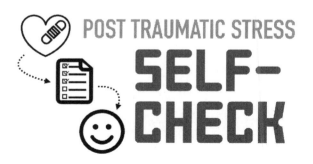

POST TRAUMATIC STRESS SELF-CHECK

Have you ever experienced any of these? According the U.S. Dept. of Veteran Affairs, in order to get a diagnosis of Post Traumatic Stress one must meet the following criteria.

Instructions: Walk through the list and check any that apply to you.

☐ **Criterion 1 (one required):** The person was exposed to: death, threatened death, actual or threatened serious injury, or actual or threatened sexual violence, in the following way(s):

- Direct exposure

- Witnessing the trauma

- Learning that a relative or close friend was exposed to a trauma

- Indirect exposure to aversive details of the trauma, usually in the course of professional duties (e.g., first responders, medics)

☐ **Criterion 2 (one required):** The traumatic event is persistently re-experienced, in the following way(s):

- Unwanted upsetting memories

- Nightmares

- Flashbacks

- Emotional distress after exposure to traumatic reminders

- Physical reactivity after exposure to traumatic reminders

☐ **Criterion 3 (one required):** Avoidance of trauma-related stimuli after the trauma, in the following way(s):

- Trauma-related thoughts or feelings

- Trauma-related reminders

- **Criterion 4 (two required):** Negative thoughts or feelings that began or worsened after the trauma, in the following way(s):

- Inability to recall key features of the trauma

- Overly negative thoughts and assumptions about oneself or the world

- Exaggerated blame of self or others for causing the trauma

- Negative affect

- Decreased interest in activities

- Feeling isolated

- Difficulty experiencing positive affect

☐ **Criterion 5 (two required):** Trauma-related arousal and reactivity that began or worsened after the trauma, in the following way(s):

- Irritability or aggression

- Risky or destructive behavior

- Hyper-vigilance

- Heightened startle reaction

- Difficulty concentrating

- Difficulty sleeping

☐ **Criterion 6 (required):** Symptoms last for more than 1 month.

☐ **Criterion 7 (required):** Symptoms create distress or functional impairment (e.g., social, occupational).

☐ **Criterion 8 (required):** Symptoms are *not* due to medication, substance use, or other illness.

☐ **Two Specifications:**

☐ **Dissociative Specification.** In addition to meeting criteria for diagnosis, an individual experiences high levels of either of the following in reaction to trauma-related stimuli:

   • **Depersonalization.** Experience of being an outside observer of or detached from oneself (e.g., feeling as if "this is not happening to me," as if one were in a dream).

   • **Derealization.** Experience of unreality, distance, or distortion (e.g., "things are not real").

☐ **Delayed Specification.** Full diagnostic criteria are not met until at least six months after the trauma(s), although onset of symptoms may occur immediately.

How many of the eight Criterion did you check? ___

Did the Two Specifications apply? Which one(s)?

Resources

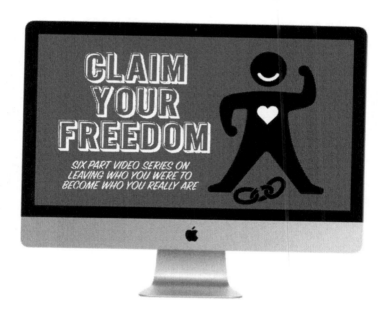

To watch the companion videos to this book, go to OilyApp.com/Freedom. Sometimes you've got to let go of who you were in order to become who you're designed to be. This book + the video series provide you with tools to do just that.

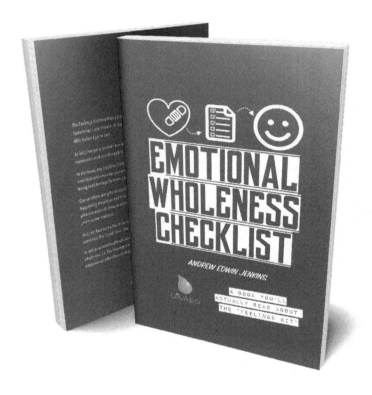

Emotional Wholeness Checklist discusses the importance of feelings. And, it provide you with a tool to manage your emotions and allow them to serve you rather than find yourself hijacked by them. Learn more at OilyApp.com/Feelings, go to OilyApp.com/books, or search amazon.com.

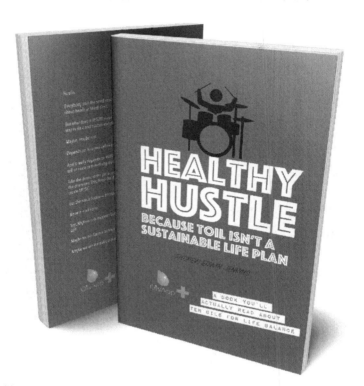

Healthy Hustle gets raw and real about why we tend to overexert ourselves: identity. A companion to *Emotional Wholeness Checklist* and *Claim Your Freedom*, this book discusses how to own who we are and then live from on overflow of a healthy soul rather than looking outside ourselves to fill those emotional reserves. Go to OilyApp.com/HealthyHustle for more info.

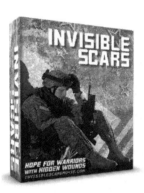 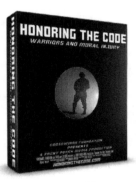

POST TRAUMATIC STRESS   MORAL INJURY

Stream the films designed specifically for veterans dealing with Post Traumatic Stress and/or Moral Injury at InvisibleScars.online. The videos and the bonus features are free.

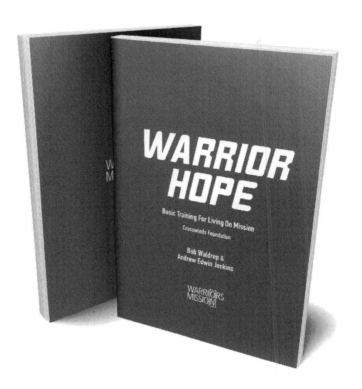

Warrior Hope takes veterans through similar concepts taught in this book. But, they are viewed from a distinctive military perspective. More info at WarriorHope.com

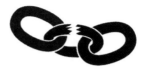

The wisest man who ever lived wrote, "There's a time for everything... a time to weep and a time to dance, a time to laugh and a time to mourn" (Ecclesiastes 3:4).

None of use are immune to hard things. And, that tough stuff might come as a one-off event, or it might come as a protracted season in which something difficult just seems to drip, drop, and dredge upon us. Rest assured, though, we all face it. In other words, it's not a matter of "if," it's a matter of "when."

The first thing to do when facing trials is to seek rest. In particular, sleep is when our bodies and our souls recover. In the same way electronic devices sometimes need a hard reset, so also do we.

You've probably seen a toddler "go bananas." Rather than scold them for being "emotional," we simply tell them, "Hey, let's get you some sleep." We know that when they rest, they'll restart fresh and anew.

Adults are the same way. And, in fact, this "rest thing" is built into the fabric of Creation. It's how the universe works.

Young Living suggests you use the Freedom Sleep kit for 30 days, followed by the Freedom Release kit. We walk through both in this book. Whereas one encourages your body, your mind, and your emotions to reset, the other enlivens you to move forward in heath and wholeness- letting go of the past and moving forward.

You'll see that we don't simply "get over" the hard things. Rather, we learn to set them in their proper place and "get through" them. Emotional wholeness isn't just about moving through the past, it's also about moving into your future.

Made in the USA
Lexington, KY
24 November 2019